Maria Strohbusch

**Neospora caninum: Killing the Survival Artist**

Maria Strohbusch

# Neospora caninum: Killing the Survival Artist

## New Treatment and Detection Approaches

Südwestdeutscher Verlag für Hochschulschriften

**Impressum/Imprint (nur für Deutschland/ only for Germany)**
Bibliografische Information der Deutschen Nationalbibliothek: Die Deutsche Nationalbibliothek verzeichnet diese Publikation in der Deutschen Nationalbibliografie; detaillierte bibliografische Daten sind im Internet über http://dnb.d-nb.de abrufbar.

Alle in diesem Buch genannten Marken und Produktnamen unterliegen warenzeichen-, marken- oder patentrechtlichem Schutz bzw. sind Warenzeichen oder eingetragene Warenzeichen der jeweiligen Inhaber. Die Wiedergabe von Marken, Produktnamen, Gebrauchsnamen, Handelsnamen, Warenbezeichnungen u.s.w. in diesem Werk berechtigt auch ohne besondere Kennzeichnung nicht zu der Annahme, dass solche Namen im Sinne der Warenzeichen- und Markenschutzgesetzgebung als frei zu betrachten wären und daher von jedermann benutzt werden dürften.

Verlag: Südwestdeutscher Verlag für Hochschulschriften Aktiengesellschaft & Co. KG
Dudweiler Landstr. 99, 66123 Saarbrücken, Deutschland
Telefon +49 681 37 20 271-1, Telefax +49 681 37 20 271-0
Email: info@svh-verlag.de
Zugl.: Bern, Universität Bern, Dissertation, 2008

Herstellung in Deutschland:
Schaltungsdienst Lange o.H.G., Berlin
Books on Demand GmbH, Norderstedt
Reha GmbH, Saarbrücken
Amazon Distribution GmbH, Leipzig
ISBN: 978-3-8381-1268-8


**Imprint (only for USA, GB)**
Bibliographic information published by the Deutsche Nationalbibliothek: The Deutsche Nationalbibliothek lists this publication in the Deutsche Nationalbibliografie; detailed bibliographic data are available in the Internet at http://dnb.d-nb.de.

Any brand names and product names mentioned in this book are subject to trademark, brand or patent protection and are trademarks or registered trademarks of their respective holders. The use of brand names, product names, common names, trade names, product descriptions etc. even without a particular marking in this works is in no way to be construed to mean that such names may be regarded as unrestricted in respect of trademark and brand protection legislation and could thus be used by anyone.

Publisher: Südwestdeutscher Verlag für Hochschulschriften Aktiengesellschaft & Co. KG
Dudweiler Landstr. 99, 66123 Saarbrücken, Germany
Phone +49 681 37 20 271-1, Fax +49 681 37 20 271-0
Email: info@svh-verlag.de

Printed in the U.S.A.
Printed in the U.K. by (see last page)
ISBN: 978-3-8381-1268-8


Copyright © 2010 by the author and Südwestdeutscher Verlag für Hochschulschriften Aktiengesellschaft & Co. KG and licensors
All rights reserved. Saarbrücken 2010

# Table of contents

*Table of contents* ............................................................................................................ *I*

*Abstract* ...................................................................................................................... *III*

*Introduction* .................................................................................................................. *1*

    1.   *Neospora caninum*: a general introduction ................................................ 1
    **1.1.**   **Parasite stages** ........................................................................................ 1
    **1.2.**   **Life cycle** ................................................................................................. 3
    **1.2.1.**   **Transmission** ....................................................................................... 4
    **1.3.**   **Neosporosis** ........................................................................................... 5
    **1.3.1.**   **Neosporosis in dogs** ........................................................................... 5
    **1.3.2.**   **Neosporosis in cattle** ........................................................................... 5
    **1.3.3.**   **Epidemiology** ....................................................................................... 7
    **1.4.**   **Detection methods** ................................................................................. 8
    **1.5.**   **NcGRA2** ................................................................................................. 9
    2.   The murine model of *N. caninum* infection ............................................. 11
    **2.1.**   **Immune response in mice during *N. caninum* infection** ..................... 12
    **2.1.1.**   **Immune response in non-pregnant mice** ......................................... 12
    **2.1.2.**   **Immune response in pregnant mice** ................................................. 13
    **2.2.**   **Vertical transmission of *N. caninum*** ................................................. 14
    3.   Treatment ................................................................................................ 15
    **3.1.**   **Treatment of cattle** ............................................................................... 15
    **3.1.1.**   **Vaccination** ........................................................................................ 15
    **3.1.2.**   **Chemotherapy** ................................................................................... 15
    **3.2.**   **Treatment of experimentally infected mice** ......................................... 16
    **3.2.1.**   **Vaccination** ........................................................................................ 16
    **3.2.2.**   **Chemotherapy** ................................................................................... 18
    **3.2.2.1.**   **Toltrazuril** ......................................................................................... 18
    4.   The immune system of newborn mice ..................................................... 21
    5.   Dendritic cells .......................................................................................... 22
    **5.1.**   **DCs and intracellular parasites** ............................................................ 23

*Summary of publications* ........................................................................................... *25*

1. NcGRA2 as a molecular target to assess the parasiticidal activity of toltrazuril against *Neospora caninum*. Strohbusch M., Müller N., Hemphill A., Greif G. and Gottstein B. (2008). Parasitology; Aug 135(9); 1065-73..................................................25

2. NcGRA2-RT-PCR to detect live versus dead parasites in *Neospora caninum*-infected mice. Strohbusch M., Müller N., Hemphill A., Greif G. and Gottstein B. (2008). The Open Parasitology Journal; in press ............................................................25

3. Toltrazuril treatment of congenitally acquired *Neospora caninum*-infection in newborn mice. Strohbusch M., Müller N., Hemphill A., Greif G. and Gottstein B. (manuscript)..................................................................................................................26

4. Survival of *Neospora caninum* inside mouse bone marrow-derived dendritic cells and induction of cytokine expression. Strohbusch M., Müller N., Hemphill A., Margos M., Grandgirard D., Greif G. and Gottstein B. (manuscript)..........................................26

*Accepted publication* ............................................................................................ 28

*Manuscripts* ........................................................................................................... 53

*Discussion* ............................................................................................................. 98

*Perspectives* ........................................................................................................ 101

*References* .......................................................................................................... 103

# Abstract

The main problem associated with *Neospora caninum* and the corresponding disease, neosporosis, are abortions in cattle causing serious veterinary health issues and economic losses within livestock production. Although, there are successful experimental vaccination approaches to prevent cerebral neosporosis or vertical transmission in mice, currently no valuable vaccines are available to protect cattle from abortion. Toltrazuril, a symmetric triazinone derivative, was shown to exhibit anti-coccidial activity against cyst-forming and non-cyst-forming coccidians. Furthermore, initially explorative approaches indicated a basic effectiveness of toltrazuril against experimental *N. caninum* infection in mice and calves. So far, efficacy of experimental treatment and vaccination *in vitro* or *in vivo* has been determined upon use of morphological criteria of affected parasites, differential demonstration of the absence or presence of parasite-induced lesions, and PCR-based detection of parasite genomicDNA (gDNA). However, the presence of parasite gDNA does not necessarily provide information on parasite viability, and conventional *in vivo* and *in vitro* tests are being used by inoculating appropriate samples into laboratory animals or cell culture.

In the work presented here, the efficacy of toltrazuril was further investigated using two approaches: (I) a mouse model to assess the effect of the drug on congenitally acquired *N. caninum*-infection in newborn mice and (II) cell culture-based assays to assess treatment duration time for parasitostatic and parasiticidal activity. Furthermore, the work was directed to establish a novel molecular detection method to clearly distinguish between live and dead parasites after a given treatment *in vitro* and *in vivo*.

For the treatment of congenitally infected pups, pregnant wild-type C57Bl/6 mice were infected at gestation day 13 and let give birth without any medication. Newborn mice were treated either with toltrazuril or the corresponding placebo at day three and four of birth. A group of newborn mice were again treated 10 and 25 days later, as another part of the study indicated a parasiticidal activity of toltrazuril after 14 days of treatment. These repeated treatments had no negative effect on the newborns as non-infected treated pups developed normal without differences in mortality and morbidity. Already one application of toltrazuril was able to delay the outbreak of neosporosis in newborn mice significantly. Survival rates were significantly higher in toltrazuril-treated pups compared to placebo-treated pups. The number of diseased and *Neospora*-positive pups was markedly reduced after the three-time-toltrazuril-treatment compared to all other groups. The three-time-treatment also resulted in the highest antibody response. The results presented in this study indicated that the treatment with three applications of toltrazuril had the best positive effect to control the course of infection in congenitally *N. caninum*-infected newborn mice.

To assess the antiparasitic activity of toltrazuril, a novel molecular detection method was built up by addressing parasite mRNA as a target to demonstrate viability or non-viability of organisms. Live parasites can be detected by measuring the mRNA level of specific genes, making use of the specific mRNA available in live cells. The *NcGra2* gene of *N. caninum*, which is known to be expressed in both tachyzoites and bradyzoites, was used to establish a quantitative real-time RT-PCR, for monitoring and quantification of viable parasites. Conventional RT-PCR was used to examine species specificity and sensitivity. NcGRA2-RT-PCR was specific for *Neospora* tachyzoites from different strains and sensitive enough to detected 0.1 parasite equivalent per reaction.

Validation of the NcGRA2-RT-PCR *in vitro* was achieved in *Neospora*-infected cells that were treated for 2 to 20 days with 30 µg/ml toltrazuril. Quantitative RT-PCR demonstrated that a 10-day-toltrazuril-treatment exerts a parasitostatic activity, as assessed by the presence of *NcGRA2*-transcripts, whereas after a 14-day-treatment period no *NcGRA2*-transcripts were detected, showing that the parasites were not viable anymore. Concurrently, further culture for a period of 4 weeks in the absence of the drug following the 14 days toltrazuril treatment did not lead to any parasite proliferation anymore, confirming the parasiticidal effect of the treatment. This assay has a potential to be widely used in the development of novel drugs against *N. caninum*, in view to distinguish between parasiticidal and parasitostatic efficacy of given compounds.

NcGRA2-RT-PCR was further adapted to detect live parasites in tissue of *Neospora*-infected mice. Organs from mice were examined 6 and 12 days post infection for containing viable parasites. Viability was proven with NcGRA2-RT-PCR and inoculation of diagnostic specimen into cell culture. Although gDNA was detected 6 dpi in almost all organs, viability of the parasites by RT-PCR or growth in cell culture could not be verified in all cases. 12 dpi, gDNA was mainly found in the brains and it was confirmed by both, RT-PCR and *in vitro* cultivation, that gDNA arose from live parasites. Comparison of the two viability tests revealed that both exhibit almost the same sensitivity (6 dpi: fair agreement with kappa 0.29; 12 dpi: substantial agreement with kappa 0.8), but RT-PCR is much faster and easier to handle with less risk of contaminations compared to the *in vitro* inoculation. The NcGRA2-RT-PCR provides an useful tool of fast live parasite detection in tissue samples instead of inoculation of material and detection of parasite growth in cell culture. Furthermore, this test can be used to distinguish between live and dead parasites in infected animals after treatment- and vaccination-studies.

The last part of the thesis work concentrated on the immune response induced by *N. caninum*. To pursue this, the interaction of *N. caninum* with dendritic cells (DCs) was examined. DCs can be activated by apicomplexan parasites, like *Toxoplasma gondii*. As found by others, extracts from *T. gondii* activated DCs and stimulated IL-12 production, whereas active *T. gondii* invasion of immature DCs suppressed the ability of these cells to participate in innate immunity and to induce adaptive immune responses. Infection of immature DCs allows the parasites to disseminate from the site of infection within cells undergoing steady-state migration to draining lymphoid organs. Nothing is known so far about the invasion ability of *N. caninum* into DCs and the survival of the parasites in these cells. In the present work, electron microscopy and NcGRA2-RT-PCR were used to identify viability of parasites inside DCs. Cytokine expression was determined to answer the question of DCs suppression or activation through the parasite.

Immature mouse bone marrow-derived DCs were stimulated with treated or untreated parasites for up to 48 h. Elektron microscopy revealed that untreated parasites were able to invade and to survive in DCs. Viability was also proven with NcGRA2-RT-PCR. Furthermore, untreated parasites were able to form parasitophorous vacuoles and proliferate inside DCs. On the other hand, treated parasites were killed by the treatment and no live tachyzoites were found in the samples. Both, treated and untreated parasites were able to stimulate cytokine expression. Expression of IL-12p40, IL-10 and TNF-α was determined and quantified using RT-PCR and cytokine-ELISA, whereas the expression of IL-4 was below detection limit. This first approach demonstrated that *N. caninum* has the ability to interact with DCs and to survive in these immune cells. In addition, live and inactivated parasites stimulated cytokine expression. Further work is now ongoing to find out whether DCs also promote dissemination of parasites throughout the host body and how *Neospora*-infected DCs influence immune system.

# Introduction

## 1. *Neospora caninum*: a general introduction

*Neospora caninum* is an obligate intracellular parasite of the family Sarcocystidae and placed as a sister group of *Toxoplasma gondii* in the phylum of Apicomplexa (Ellis et al., 1994). *N. caninum* was first identified in 1984 in dogs with encephalomyelitis and myositis (Bjerkas et al., 1984). Infection with *N. caninum* leads to a disease named neosporosis, which primarily affects dogs and cattle with the consequences of neurological disorder. However, most importantly, the current evidence strongly indicates that *N. caninum* is the protozoan pathogen most commonly associated with bovine abortion worldwide. Therefore, infection of cattle with *N. caninum* represents an important veterinary health problem and is of high economical significance. It is not yet known how cattle initially become infected in nature. At least, infection within a herd occurs through vertical transmission during pregnancy of infected dams. So far, there is no treatment available preventing cattle from neosporosis.

### 1.1. Parasite stages

To date, three infectious stages have been identified in the life cycle of *N. caninum*. These are tachyzoites, bradyzoites within tissue cysts and sporozoites within oocysts. Tachyzoites and bradyzoites are the obligate intracellular, asexual stages of the parasite, found in both intermediate and definitive hosts. Oocysts are the result of the sexual cycle, taking place only in the intestine of definitive hosts.

Tachyzoites (Fig. 1A) are ovoid, lunate or globular and are 7.5 x 2 µm in size (Speer et al., 1999). They are able to infect a wide range of cell types, including fibroblasts, vascular endothelial cells, epidermal keratinocytes, macrophages, natural killer cells and neural cells (Boysen et al., 2006; Hemphill et al., 1996; Pinheiro et al., 2006; Vonlaufen et al., 2002), suggesting a low host cell specificity (Hemphill et al., 1999). Within the host cell cytoplasm, tachyzoites are enclosed in a parasitophorous vacuole. They proliferate by endodyogeny (internal budding), producing hundreds of new parasites within a few days. Rapidly dividing tachyzoites form a pseudocyst, which is lacking a cyst wall. After the pseudocyst reaches a critical mass, host cell lysis occurs and the freshly egressed tachyzoites can infect new neighbouring cells or disseminate throughout the body. The host immune system is one of the factors that trigger the conversion of tachyzoites into bradyzoites (Buxton et al., 2002).

Bradyzoites (Fig. 1B) are slender and slightly longer than tachyzoites, measuring 8.1 x 2 µm (Speer et al., 1999). They represent a slowly dividing stage of the parasite, capable to form tissue cysts containing up to 100 bradyzoites. Tissue cysts are round to oval in shape and up to 100 µm long. They are surrounded by a 1-4 µm thick cyst wall, depending on how long the infection has existed (Dubey et al., 2002). The cysts wall provides a chemically and physiologically stable environment and allows the parasite to persist for several years within an immuno-competent host. However, in an immuno-compromised situation, such as pregnancy, bradyzoites can get reactivated and transform back into tachyzoites (Rettigner et al., 2004). Tissue cysts are mostly located in the central nervous system (Dubey and Lindsay, 1996), but were also found in skeletal muscles of both intermediate and definitive hosts (Peters et al., 2001).

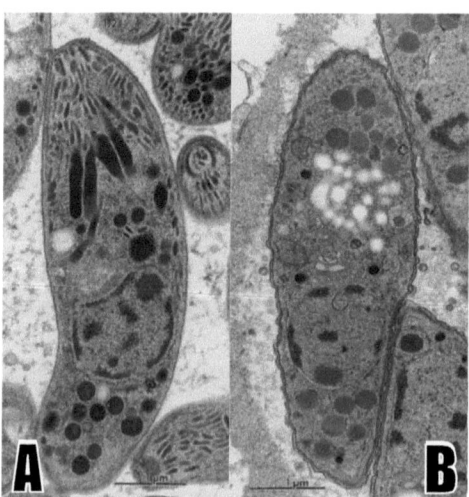

Figure 1: Transmission EM of *N. caninum* (A) tachyzoites and (B) bradyzoites (Speer et al., 1999).

Oocysts (Fig. 2) are spherical to subspherical, approximately 11 µm in diameter and surrounded by a smooth, colourless and 0.6-0.8 µm thick oocyst wall (Lindsay et al.,

1999). Unsporulated oocysts (Fig. 2A) are produced during sexual development in the intestine of definitive hosts und shed in their faeces. The schizogenic and gametogenic stages that are presumed to precede the formation of oocysts have not yet been observed, but sporulation of oocysts in the environment was found to result in orally infectious oocysts containing two sporocysts with four sporozoites each (McAllister et al., 1998). Sporulated oocysts (Fig. 2B) remain infective after the storage at 4°C in 2% sulphuric acid for up to 108 days (Gondim et al., 2004).

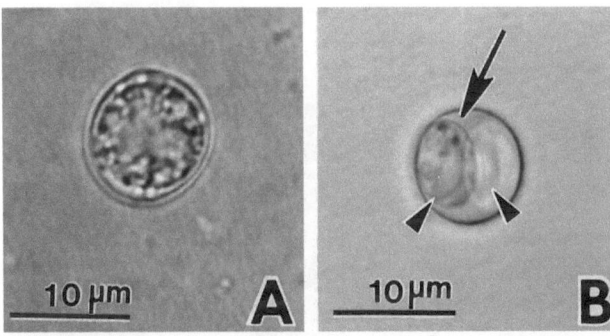

Figure 2: (A) unsporulated oocyst, (B) sporulated oocyst with two sporocysts (arrow) and with sporozoites (arrowheads) (McAllister et al., 1998).

## 1.2. Life cycle

The life cycle (Fig. 3) of *N. caninum* consists of an asexual and a sexual cycle. The asexual cycle occurs in intermediate and definitive hosts, whereas the sexual cycle occurs in definitive hosts only. Dogs and coyotes have been identified as definitive hosts (Gondim et al., 2004; McAllister et al., 1998). Cattle and a wide range of other ruminant animals, such as goats and sheep, can act as intermediate hosts (Dubey, 2003). A sylvatic cycle is proposed, occurring between coyotes and white-tailed deer (Gondim, 2006). Recently, also chicken (*Gallus domesticus*) were found to be natural intermediate hosts of *N. caninum* (Costa et al., 2008).

Definitive hosts can acquire infection by consumption of *N. caninum* infected tissue (Gondim et al., 2002; Lindsay et al., 1999). Within the canine intestinal tissue sexual multiplication takes place, followed by shedding of unsporulated oocysts in the faeces. After consumption of food or water contaminated with oocysts through intermediate hosts, oocysts excyst in the small intestine and release sporozoites. In the intestinal epithelium, sporozoites transform into tachyzoites. These tachyzoites are then released into the blood, resulting in dissemination of the parasite throughout the host body (Dubey et al., 2006). Tachyzoites invade different tissues and multiply asexually rapidly. With the onset of the host immune response, tachyzoites revert into bradyzoites and form tissue cysts.

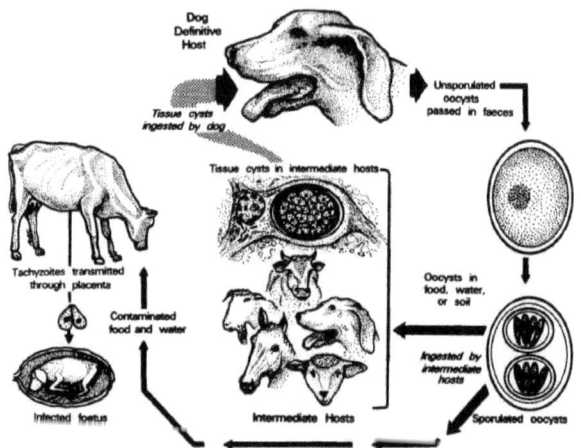

Figure 3: Life cycle of *N. caninum*, including definitive and intermediate hosts (Dubey, 1999).

### 1.2.1. Transmission

Horizontal and vertical transmission are the two main routes of *N. caninum* infection. Horizontal transmission occurs postnatally through the ingestion of oocysts or tissue cysts. Vertical transmission, also called transplacental or congenital transmission, occurs by transmission of parasites from an infected pregnant mother to her foetus. Recently, it was proposed to use the terms `endogenous` and `exogenous` transplacental transmission (Fig. 4) as a more precise alternative to such inadequate terms as `vertical` or `congenital` (Trees and Williams, 2005). In a persistently infected dam, recrudescence of the infection led to an endogenous transplacental tramsission of the parasite to the foetus (Rettigner et al., 2004). Exogenous transplancental transmission was shown to take place when a naïve pregnant dam becomes infected through the consumption of oocysts (Gondim et al., 2004; McCann et al., 2007). Transplancental transmission seems to be the main route of infection for cattle and spread of the parasite within the herd.

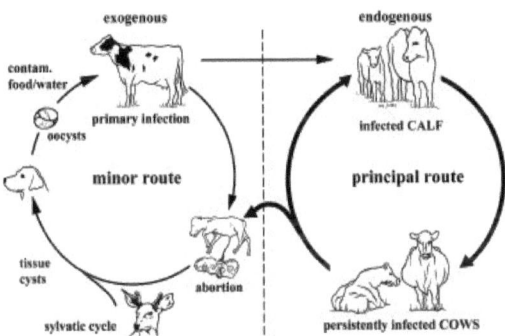

Figure 4: Exogenous and endogenous transplacental infection in cattle (Dubey et al., 2006).

## 1.3. Neosporosis

### 1.3.1. Neosporosis in dogs

*N. caninum* causes serious diseases in dogs, including encephalitis and myositis (Bjerkas et al., 1984). Dogs of any age developed clinical signs, which were either generalized or localized (Barber and Trees, 1996). A subclinically infected bitch transmitted the parasite to her foetuses, and successive litters may were born infected (Dubey et al., 1990; Dubey and Lindsay, 1989). The most severe cases of disease occured in young, congenitally infected pups, which showed an initial hind limb paresis that progresses to paralysis (Dubey et al., 1988; Patitucci et al., 1997). Cutaneous neosporosis was also observed in immunosuppressed or older aminals (Dubey et al., 1988; Perl et al., 1998). Anti-protozoal drugs, including clindamycin, sulfonamides and pyrimethamine, were used to treat neosporosis in dogs (Barber and Trees, 1996; Dubey et al., 1998).

### 1.3.2. Neosporosis in cattle

*N. caninum* has become of international concern owing to the connection of infection by this parasite with abortion in dairy and beef cattle. Infected adult cattle do not exhibit clinical signs of disease. The only manifestations of infection in a pregnant animal are: (I) abortion of the foetus or embryo; (II) birth of a weak calf; (III) or delivery of a clinically healthy but persistently infected calf, depending on the gestational age (Dubey and Lindsay, 1996; Quinn et al., 2002; Williams et al., 2000). Congenitally infected heifers transmitted the parasite to their own offspring later (Björkman et al., 1996). Nevertheless, a recent study showed that the infection has also an economic impact, in that milk production in first-lactation dairy cows was significantly reduced (Thurmond and Hietala, 1997). Neosporosis-induced abortions occured year-round (Dubey, 2003) and were epidemic, endemic or sporadic. Cows of any age may abort from 3 month gestation to term, but most of the abortions occur at 5-6 month gestation. Sero-positive cows were more likely to abort than sero-negative cows (Sager et al., 2001; Wouda et al., 1998). Maternal antibodies acquired during a first gestation did not prevent foetal infection in subsequent gestations and, perhaps, did not prevent maternal re-infection (Piergili Fioretti et al., 2000). Persistently infected cattle had an immune response that did not protect against recrudescence, but protected against exogenous challenge infection (Williams and Trees, 2006). It was also shown that *N. caninum* infection can be maintained over several bovine generations and that recrudescing persistent infection, rather than a new infection, explains *Neospora* infection of calves (Piergili Fioretti et al., 2003). When *N. caninum* invaded cells in the bovine uterus, it multiplied and caused focal destruction of both maternal and foetal tissue at the maternal-foetal interface, as well as initiation of an inflammatory response (Macaldowie et al., 2004; Maley et al., 2003). From there, the damage extended out into the chorioallantois (the foetal placental membranes) between the cotyledons and at the same time, parasites entered the foetal bloodstream and invaded further tissues, with a predilection for the CNS (Buxton et al., 2002).

Infection with *N. caninum* oocysts during pregnancy resulted in exogenous transplacental infection of the foetus. Thereby the risk of foetal infection was affected by two important factors: the number of oocysts and the time of pregnancy when the oocysts are consumed (McCann et al., 2007). The risk of transplacental transmission increased at later times of exposure and with larger doses of oocysts. Experimental inoculation of cattle at day 70 of gestation with *N. caninum* tachyzoites caused foetal death, with parasite-associated lesions in the placenta and foetus (Macaldowie et al., 2004). Further investigation with naturally infected animals showed that the risk period for abortion was beyond 90 days of pregnancy (Lopez-Gatius et al., 2004). Infection of pregnant heifers at gestation day 120 resulted, among different IFN-$\gamma$ levels, in a predominant IgG2 response, a mixed IgG1/IgG2 response as well as a predominant IgG1 response, whereas the infected foetuses mounted strong *N. caninum*-specific humoral responses, with a predominant IgG1 response (Andrianarivo et al., 2001). However, cell-mediated immune responses

(IFN-γ levels) were highly variable between foetuses, suggesting that the full development of cell-mediated immune responses in bovine foetuses might occur at more variable periods in gestation than humoral responses (Bartley et al., 2004). Factors influencing the outcome of *N. caninum* infection in pregnancy include: (I) the timing, quantity and duration of parasitaemia during gestation; (II) the effectiveness of the maternal immune response; and (III) the ability of the foetus to mount an effective immune response (Innes et al., 2005). The foetal immune system is an extremely important factor in the pathogenesis of *N. caninum*. In the third trimester of gestation, mature foetuses were sufficiently immunocompetent to limit parasite multiplication, to control infection and to survive (Piergili Fioretti et al., 2000).

### 1.3.3. Epidemiology

Worldwide, many species of mammals have been exposed to *N. caninum*. Data of different epidemiological studies were not comparable due to different serologic methods and cut-off values used, as well as being based on convenience samples obtained for other purposes (Dubey et al., 2007).

None or only a few seropositive dogs were found on the Falkland Islands, in Kenya or in Sweden (Barber et al., 1997; Björkman et al., 1994). On the other hand, up to 100% seropositive dogs were observed on farms in New Zealand (Antony and Williamson, 2003). In Switzerland 7.3% pet dogs and 20% dairy farm dogs were shown to have antibodies against *N. caninum* (Sager et al., 2006). Seroprevalence of *N. caninum* antibodies in dairy cattle ranged from 1.3% in Sweden (Bartels et al., 2006) to 64.5% in Argentina (Venturini et al., 1999). In beef cattle *N. caninum* antibodies were present in 1.5% of the Japanese beef cattle (Koiwai et al., 2005) and in up to 79% in some herds from the United States (McAllister et al., 2000). A swiss case control study detected *Neospora* antibodies in 44% of all aborting cows (Sager et al., 2001). Antibodies to *N. caninum* were also found in noncanine, nonbovine domestic animals around the world, including cats, pigs, sheep and goats (Damriyasa et al., 2004; Dubey et al., 1996; Ferroglio et al., 2005; Hässig et al., 2003). In wildlife animals high prevalences of *N. caninum* were detected, for example in foxes, lions and zebras (Buxton et al., 1997; Ferroglio et al., 2003). Interestingly, *N. caninum* infections were also found in marine mammals, including sea otter, walrus or dolphins (Dubey et al., 2003).

Further on, rhesus macaques have been successfully infected with *N. caninum* (Barr et al., 1994; Ho et al., 1997), but there is no proven evidence that the parasite can also cause neosporosis-like disease in humans, although anti-*Neospora caninum* antibodies were detected in both immuno-compromised and healthy people (Lobato et al., 2006; Nam et al., 1998; Tranas et al., 1999). In a recent study in England, no evidence of human exposure to *N. caninum* was found in a high-risk population, suggesting that human infection is unlikely in England (McCann et al., 2008). Nothing is known about how far *N. caninum* causes clinical signs in other mammals among dogs, cattle, sheep and goats.

Neosporosis in cattle is the most important and economically most substantial problem caused by the parasite. Financial costs were associated with abortion, premature culling and reduced milk yield (Chi et al., 2002; Thurmond and Hietala, 1996, 1997). In Switzerland, estimated economic losses for Swiss dairy producers due to *N. caninum* were calculated to be around € 9.7 million per year (Häsler et al., 2006).

## 1.4. Detection methods

There are a number of different diagnostic tools available to detect *N. caninum* and to discriminate neosporosis from infections with closely related parasites, like *Toxoplasma* and *Sarcocystis*. Indirect techniques are based on the detection of *Neospora* antibodies in the blood and include indirect fluorescence antibody test (IFAT) and enzyme-linked immunosorbent assay (ELISA). IFAT is the most widely used and most specific assay, as there is no or only little cross-reactivity with antibodies from other related parasites. The indirect methods give information about whether an individual animal is or has recently been exposed to the parasite, but they do not prove the parasite to be the causative agent. To discriminate between recent and chronic *N. caninum* infection, an IgG avidity ELISA was developed for use in cattle (Björkman et al., 1999).

Direct detection techniques include microscopic methods, polymerase chain reaction (PCR) and *in vitro* isolation of the parasite. *N. caninum* tachyzoites and tissue cysts can directly be identified by immunofluorescence techniques using fluorescence microscopy. Histopathological lesions induced by parasites are already visible with light microscopy, but in order to confirm neosporosis, the causative agent has to be detected in such lesions. In the last few years, diagnosis of neosporosis has been much improved by the development of *N. caninum*-specific PCRs, which allow highly sensitive and specific detection of the parasite (Kaufmann et al., 1996; Müller et al., 2001; Müller et al., 1996). Commonly used PCRs amplify specific sequences, such as the internal transcribed spacer 1 (ITS 1) (Payne and Ellis, 1996) or a *Neospora*-specific genomic DNA (gDNA) sequence named Nc5 (Kaufmann et al., 1996). The conventional Nc5-PCR was adapted to diagnostic operating standard by introduction of the uracil DNA glycosidase (UDG) system, which eliminates potential carry-over contaminations of amplified target DNA from previous reactions (Müller et al., 1996). The same PCR was improved later for specific quantification of DNA amplification products by hybridization of Nc5-specific fluorescence-labelled detection probes and using the LightCycler instrument (Vonlaufen et al., 2002). Nowadays, quantification of parasites is a useful tool to study parasite distribution and load in tissue, blood or semen of infected animals (Collantes-Fernàndez et al., 2006; Collantes-Fernàndez et al., 2002; Ferre et al., 2005), but also to examine proliferation, adhesion and invasion probability of the parasite in cell culture after treatment (Esposito et al., 2005; Naguleswaran et al., 2003).

However, the presence of parasite gDNA or antigens in infected tissue did not necessarily provide information on parasite viability, and conventional *in vivo* and *in vitro* tests were used by inoculation of appropriate samples into laboratory animals or cell culture (Dubey et al., 2007). Immunosuppressed mice, IFN-γ knock-out mice and Mongolian jirds (*Meriones unguiculatus*) are highly susceptible to *N. caninum* and were therefore used for inoculation of infected material (Dubey et al., 1998; Dubey and Lindsay, 2000; Ramamoorthy et al., 2005). The success of these methods strongly depends on the number of parasites and the state of the tissues. Especially in cell culture, opportunistic microbial contaminations are a severe problem, as cultures have to be observed for a long time period.

### 1.5. NcGRA2

Although the genome of *N. caninum* is not yet fully described, several genes could be identified by comparison with the related parasite *Toxoplasma gondii*. Immunoscreening of a cDNA library derived from mRNA of *N. caninum* tachyzoites resulted in the identification of a clone with a deduced protein sequence exhibiting significant homology to the gene product of the 28 kDa (GRA2) antigen of *T. gondii* (Ellis et al., 2000). In *T. gondii*, the *TgGra2* gene product is an excreted-secreted antigen, which is stored in dense granules and secreted into the parasitophorous vacuole after host cell invasion (Mercier et al.,

1993). Since the corresponding mRNA was abundantly present in *N. caninum* tachyzoites, it was assumed that the gene is highly expressed in this stage (Ellis et al., 2000). The *TgGra2* gene of *T. gondii* was found to be constitutively expressed in both, tachyzoites and bradyzoites (Manger et al., 1998). Recently, it was shown that the *N. caninum NcGRA2* gene was threefold overexpressed in tachyzoites compared to bradyzoites (Kang et al., 2008). The NcGRA2 protein was found to be associated with the parasitophorous tubular network in tachyzoites and incorporated into the cyst wall of *in vitro* derived bradyzoites (Vonlaufen et al., 2004).

## 2. The murine model of *N. caninum* infection

Cattle, the natural hosts, are inappropriate for large-scale experiments. For various questions, the cheaper and easier handle murine model of *N. caninum* infection is used. Because of the short gestation period of mice compared with cattle (21 days versus 9 months), it is possible to complete several experiments regarding vertical transmission in a relatively short time frame. Furthermore, it is possible to use larger numbers of animals to generate data that can be analysed statistically. The development of clinical neosporosis depends on the mouse strain, strain and dose of parasites, treatment and way of infection (Collantes-Fernàndez et al., 2004; Lindsay and Dubey, 1989; Lindsay and Dubey, 1989; Quinn et al., 2002; Rettigner et al., 2004). Infection of mice simulated acute and chronic infection with different clinical signs and production of tissue cysts (Collantes-Fernàndez et al., 2004; Rettigner et al., 2004). One important topic is the vertical transmission, which also occurs in mice and depends on the stage of pregnancy when infection takes place (Liddell et al., 1999; Omata et al., 2004; Quinn et al., 2002; Ramamoorthy et al., 2007). Not all mouse strains appear equally susceptible to neosporosis. It is difficult to induce clinical illness in outbred mice without using immunosuppressor methylprednisolone, because they are naturally resistant to the parasite (Lindsay et al., 1995). Inbred mice are more sensitive to *N. caninum*. There were more severe cerebral lesions and higher brain parasite burdens in inbred (BALB/c) than in outbred (ICR) mice (Collantes-Fernàndez et al., 2004). Inbred C57BL/6 mice were very well suited for *N. caninum* infection studies as they not only showed clinical signs of the disease, but also transmitted the parasite to their offspring without the use of immunosuppressive agents (Ramamoorthy et al., 2007).

Another suitable model of acute neosporosis, beside the mouse model, is the Mongolian jird model. Mongolian jirds (*Meriones unguiculatus*) are more susceptible to neosporosis than are mice, resulting in clear-cut results. The jird model can be used to screen candidate treatments and to test the efficacy of vaccines for neosporosis, but not for examination of immune mechanisms since there are no jird-specific immunological reagents available so far (Ramamoorthy et al., 2005).

## 2.1. Immune response in mice during *N. caninum* infection

The immunological response to *N. caninum* infection has not been well understood yet. Generally, the immune response to *N. caninum* infection, similar to other intracellular protozoan parasites, is dominated by a T-helper (Th) 1 cell mediated immune response. However, this is incompatible with successful pregnancy, because a Th1 response may result in non-viable offspring upon histo-incompatibility problems. The transient switch to a more Th2-oriented response supports, on the one hand, the development of the foetus, but on the other hand also yields in an increased parasite burden in the mother (Quinn et al., 2002).

There is a complex interplay between the different facets of the immune system. Early production of inflammatory cytokines is required for parasite-induced protective immune responses. However, if uncontrolled, this response can lead to severe immunopathologic changes and even death. The strength of the host cell-mediated immune response must be tightly regulated to limit the infection, and also to avoid immunopathologic changes. $CD8^+$ cells, for instance, may act primarily as cytotoxic cells during acute infection. An excess of $CD8^+$ cells, however, may exacerbate cell destruction or cytokine production, leading to more severe neurological signs (Spencer et al., 2005). Furthermore, regulatory T-cells ($CD25^+CD4^+$), triggered by initial dendritic cell (DC) activity, play a crucial role in subsequent outcome of immune orientation, influencing the course of infection (Belkaid and Oldenhove, 2008).

### 2.1.1. Immune response in non-pregnant mice

The Th1 response includes cell-mediated immunity. It is marked by significant levels of IFN-γ, IL-12, TNF-α and an IgG2a-dominant antibody response (Quinn et al., 2004).

IFN-γ may play an important role in the regulation of parasite growth in tissues. IFN-γ-knock-out mice rapidly developed acute neosporosis and died within a few days after infection (Nishikawa et al., 2001; Ritter et al., 2002). Neutralisation of IFN-γ resulted in increased mortality and severe morbidity during acute *N. caninum* infection (Baszler et al., 1999), suggesting that early IFN-γ production has a crucial role in induction of protective immune responses against *N. caninum* infection (Nishikawa et al., 2001). IFN-γ-induced parasite growth-inhibitory activity in macrophages and an increased NO production was an important mechanism for killing of intracellular *N. caninum* (Tanaka et al., 2000). However, TNF-α and inducible nitric oxide synthase (iNOS; an enzyme that produce NO) did not appear to play a critical role in acute or chronic *N. caninum* infection (Ritter et al., 2002). IL-12 decreased the severity of early clinical disease and was required for sustained stimulation of a protective Th1 immune response to *N. caninum* infection (Baszler et al., 1999). The production might be regulated by sufficient synthesis of IFN-γ (Nishikawa et al., 2001).

Antibodies may play a crucial role in the control of infection because B-cell deficient C57BL/6 (μMT) mice could not control infection and died some days post infection (Ammann et al., 2004; Eperon et al., 1999). An important characteristic of the Th1 response is the production of IgG2a. The major parasite-specific IgG subtypes displayed in sera of *Neospora*-infected mice were IgG2a and IgG2b and to a lesser extent, IgG3, whereas no IgG1 was detected (Eperon et al., 1999). A protective role of B cells can be explained by stimulation or costimulation of T-cells through CD80 or CD86 (Teixeira et al., 2005).

Further on, suitable production of Th1/Th2-type cytokines is essential for the control of parasite burdens in hosts. The IL-4-mediated regulation of IFN-γ effects might play an important role in cellular responses against parasite infection, such as activation of antigen-presenting cells and production of antibodies against the parasite (Nishikawa et al., 2003).

### 2.1.2. Immune response in pregnant mice

The Th1 response associated with infection of intracellular parasites compromises the viability of the foetus, whereas a Th2 response aids the maintenance of pregnancy. However, the Th2 response also allows parasite transmission to the foetus and compromises the health of the mother by increasing the parasite burden.

Description of systemic changes in cytokine production between pregnant and non-pregnant QS mice in response to *N. caninum* infection revealed that pregnant infected mice produced IFN-γ, IL-12 and TNF-α at levels lower than infected non-pregnant mice.

Both, infected non-pregnant and infected pregnant mice produced similar levels of IL-10, an important Th2 cytokine, whereas only infected pregnant mice showed a significant IL-4 production as a result of the combined effect of infection and pregnancy (Quinn et al., 2004). IL-4 is an inhibitor of Th1 cells and is responsible for subtype switching to IgG1.

## 2.2. Vertical transmission of *N. caninum*

Several studies pointed out that the transmission and abortion rate depend on the time point of infection of the mother during pregnancy. Infection before, or early in, pregnancy caused foetal losses in BALB/c mice, although there were no parasites detected in foetal-placental tissues (Long and Baszler, 1996). Infection of BALB/c mice between days 8 and 12 of gestation resulted in a high frequency of parasite transmission (Liddell et al., 1999). A vertical transmission rate of 100% was observed in C57BL/6 mice, infected between days 12 and 14 of pregnancy (Ramamoorthy et al., 2007). Otherwise, no reproductive loss was observed in mice infected with *N. caninum* in late stages of pregnancy (Quinn et al., 2002). Further, infection late in pregnancy had no effect on foetal viability and newborns were mostly asymptomatic, but apparently infected.

Examination of the relationship between Th1/Th2 immune response and the occurrence of vertical transmission in BALB/c mice led to the hypothesis that only very few parasites multiply and that transplacental transmission occurs without immune response, or that *N. caninum* may either suppress type 1 response or enhance type 2 response in maternal tissues (Kano et al., 2005).

# 3. Treatment

## 3.1. Treatment of cattle

### 3.1.1. Vaccination

Since several years, the development of an effective vaccine against bovine neosporosis is a highly proposed aim. Using live parasites (non-virulent or less virulent strains) as vaccines has the advantage that they are more likely to induce an appropriate cell-mediated immune response in hosts. However, they are expensive to produce, and there might be reversal to virulence. Killed parasites are generally regarded as safe vaccines. However, they are usually unable to stimulate the required cell-mediated mechanisms and can lack some of the protective antigens. A recent study demonstrated that immunization with live tachyzoites prior to pregnancy conferred 100% protection against *Neospora*-induced foetopathy in cattle, whereas immunization with tachyzoite lysate failed to confer any protection (Williams et al., 2007). Cattle experimentally inoculated with live *N. caninum* tachyzoites prior to mating developed a sufficient immunity to inhibit vertical transmission of parasites to offspring, following a further parasite challenge at mid-gestation (Innes et al., 2001). The studies also indicated that there is a significant change in maternal immune response around mid-gestation, compared to early gestation, and that the mother might be less able to cope with the *N. caninum* infection, which in a persistently infected animal might lead to recrudescence, parasitaemia and infection of the foetus. A commercial vaccine, based on whole killed tachyzoites (Bovilis® Neoguard, Intervet) is already available in the United States. After immunization with two doses of the commercial vaccine during pregnancy, the force of abortion was reduced twice in the vaccinated group, as shown in a standard field trial in Costa Rica (Romero et al., 2004).

Future challenges in vaccine design involved a fine balancing act that must allow intervention in a manner that will tip the host parasite balance in favour of the host, without compromising pregnancy (Innes et al., 2002).

### 3.1.2. Chemotherapy

First chemotherapeutical approaches in *Neospora*-infected calves were done using ponazuril and toltrazuril, of which efficacy for prevention of parasite dissemination was tested in the mouse model (Gottstein et al., 2001). The results indicated a basic effectiveness of ponazuril against experimental *N. caninum* infection in calves (Kritzner et al., 2002). Treatment of calves from *Neospora*-seropositive cows with toltrazuril mounted a strong humoral immunity, while placebo-treated animals responded weakly to the persistent infection (Haerdi et al., 2006).

## 3.2. Treatment of experimentally infected mice

The ulterior motive of most research projects on *N. caninum* is the development of effective strategies to eliminate the parasite. This must involve treatment of chronic neosporosis without clinical signs such as vertical transmission. Several attempts of vaccination have been approached (Alaeddine et al., 2005; Liddell et al., 1999; Miller et al., 2005), and also chemotherapy has been tried using infected pregnant or non-pregnant mice (Gottstein et al., 2001; Gottstein et al., 2005).

Alternatively, it was demonstrated that induction of maternal Th1 responses against *N. caninum* could prevent vertical transmission, and that modulation of Th2 cytokines, giving anti-IL-4 monoclonal antibodies before pregnancy could reduce the frequency of vertical transmission (Long and Baszler, 2000). Thus, modulation of maternal immune responses can induce immunity to congenital *N. caninum* transmission, although the effector mechanism has not been determined yet.

### 3.2.1. Vaccination

Methods for improvement of *N. caninum* vaccines require subunits directing the immune system towards specific antigens or epitopes that induce a protective response. In this regard, much research is done on *N. caninum* surface proteins in attempt to target the immune responses towards antigens accessible during the extracellular phase of parasitemia, or toward proteins crucial for parasite transmission and survival. One important vaccine candidate is the surface protein NcSRS2 (*N. caninum* SAG1 related sequence 2), which plays a role in attachment and invasion of host cells. Immunization of mice with native NcSRS2 prior to pregnancy induced protective immunity to parasite challenge given during pregnancy, which was biased to a Th2 immune response and thereby significantly reduced congenital transmission (Haldorson et al., 2005). It was shown that monoclonal antibodies against NcSRS2 reduced attachment and invasion of placental trophoblast *in vitro* (Haldorson et al., 2005; Haldorson et al., 2006). Furthermore, rhoptry proteins are most likely to play a crucial role in host cell invasion. Vaccination with the rhoptry-associated protein, NcRPO2, was recently found to mediate protection against experimental *N. caninum* infection and cerebral disease in mice, which was associated with a protective Th1- or Th2-biased immune response, depending on the adjuvant used (Debache et al., 2008). A further important group of proteins used as vaccine candidates are secretory proteins, because they are implicated in playing a key role in the physical interaction between parasites and host cells. Vaccination with recombinant immuno-dominant microneme-associated protein NcMIC3 reduced cerebral infection of *N. caninum* infected C57BL/6 mice due to a mixed Th1/Th2 (IgG1/IgG2a)-type immune response (Cannas et al., 2003). Vaccination of mice with recombinant microneme antigen NcMIC1 elicited a humoral immune response against native *N. caninum* antigen, associated with a reduced parasite burden and absence of clinical signs of cerebral neosporosis upon challenge infection (Alaeddine et al., 2005).

In addition, there are some studies that investigate the feasibility of vaccination with live or crude *N. caninum* tachyzoites to prevent vertical transfer from experimentally infected dams to their offspring. Vaccination of female BALB/c mice with a single inoculation of crude *N. caninum* tachyzoites lysate resulted in complete protection against vertical infection of offspring (Liddell et al., 1999). Injection of live, less virulent NC-Nowra tachyzoites prior to pregnancy was very effective in reducing transplacental transmission of a challenge infection (Miller et al., 2005). The advantage of this method is that live infection can stimulate both humoral and cell-mediated responses, resulting in protective immunity. The disadvantage, however, is that the animal is chronically infected. For this reason, Miller et al. (2005) determined the effect of vaccination with a crude lysate of NC-Nowra. It was shown that injection of crude lysate stimulated a strong IgG1 response that was not particularly effective at preventing transplacental transmission.

The efficacy of γ-irradiated *N. caninum* strain Nc-1 tachyzoites as a vaccine for neosporosis was assessed in C57BL/6 mice (Ramamoorthy et al., 2006). γ-irradiation arrested parasite replication, but not host cell penetration. All vaccinated mice remained healthy, whereas unvaccinated mice died after challenge with parasites.

### 3.2.2. Chemotherapy

Chemotherapy represents an interesting alternative to the highly propagated vaccination strategy. With regard to natural hosts, attempts to treat neosporosis have remained in their initial stages, and no efficient treatment strategies have been elaborated yet. So far, a wide range of compounds have been tested in cell culture-based assays and some pharmacologically active compounds, including lasalocid, monensin, piritrexim, pyrimethamine and trimethoprim, were found to exhibit parasiticidal activity against *N. caninum* (Lindsay and Dubey, 1989; Lindsay et al., 1994). In addition, artemisinin and depudecin inhibited intracellular multiplication of *N. caninum* tachyzoite in cell culture (Kim et al., 2002; Kwon et al., 2003). More recently, it was reported that nitazoxanide (NTZ) and a series of NTZ-derivatives efficiently inhibited *N. caninum* proliferation (Esposito et al., 2007; Esposito et al., 2006; Esposito et al., 2005). NTZ is known to exhibit a broad spectrum of activity against a wide variety of intestinal parasites and enteric bacteria. The results indicated that NTZ treatment exerts true parasiticidal activity after 5 days of treatment, resulting in inhibition of *N. caninum* proliferation and severe damage of tachyzoites, but host cells were also involved (Esposito et al., 2005). Further studies are required to investigate whether NTZ or derivatives are useful for *in vivo* treatment of *N. caninum* infections. Novel diamidine compounds were found to exhibit *in vitro* activity against *N. caninum* and *T. gondii* in the submicromolar range, rendering these parasite-specific compounds promising candidates for further *in vivo* studies (Leepin et al., 2008). *In vivo* studies using oral drug treatment of *Neospora*-infected mice with sulfadiazine and amprolium pointed out that 14 days of treatment with 1 mg/ml sulfadiazine in drinking water was needed to protect 90% of infected mice, whereas amprolium at the same concentration had no effect (Lindsay and Dubey, 1990).

#### 3.2.2.1. Toltrazuril

Toltrazuril, a symmetrical triazinone compound, primarily inhibits the transfer of electrons along the respiratory chain of chloroplast like organelles, as for instance the apicoplast, and secondarily, it also affects two enzymes of pyrimidine synthesis (Harder and Haberkorn, 1989). Toltrazuril is a weak acid compound (p$K_a$ 6.8) with high lipid solubility and as such, expected to penetrate blood brain barrier reasonably well. Cerebrospinal fluid and serum concentrations of toltrazuril were assessed in horses after oral dosing (Furr and Kennedy, 2000). Results of this study indicated that toltrazuril is well-absorbed in horses.

Further, results confirmed accumulation of toltrazuril and its metabolites within cerebrospinal fluid and serum of horses after oral dosing.

Toltrazuril in combination with vaccination might be an alternative approach to an improved coccidiosis control (Greif, 2000). In cell culture-based assays, the effects of toltrazuril against *N. caninum* were tested (Darius et al., 2004). The results of this study pointed out that low concentration of the drug lead to reduction in the multiplication rate of the parasites. This effect, and especially the morphological damage at the level of apicoplasts and mitochondria, increased with rising dosages of the drug. At a high concentration, the severity of the effects was time dependent, but also cytotoxic for host cells. All in all, the damage of tachyzoites was so severe even at low concentrations that it can be considered lethal.

Toltrazuril treatment does not interfere with the development of a parasite-specific immune response. For the apicomplexan parasite *Eimeria falciformis* it was shown that toltrazuril treatment and thereby abbreviation of primary infection did not affect the development of protective immunity against challenge infection (Steinfelder et al., 2005). A study was undertaken to answer the question, whether a humoral or cellular immune response is required to support chemotherapy with toltrazuril (Ammann et al., 2004). The group demonstrated that, although antibodies may play a crucial role in the control of infection, toltrazuril seems to be efficient in reducing the dissemination of tachyzoites even in the absence of antibodies. On the other hand, a parasitostatic effect of toltrazuril was shown that required the accompaniment of T-cell immunity to evoke its full effect. However, it was indicated that 6-day toltrazuril treatment had a parasitostatic rather than a parasiticidal effect.

Chemotherapy, using either toltrazuril or ponazuril (toltrazuril sulfone), both applied in a drinking-water formulation, completely prevented the formation of cerebral lesions in experimentally infected C57BL/6 mice and resulted in a lower antibody response compared to non-treated mice (Gottstein et al., 2001). Treatment with toltrazuril also eliminated the parasite in infected BALB/c mice, while treatment with ponazuril resulted in a remanifestion of symptoms of chronic neosporosis (Darius et al., 2004).

A further work concentrated on the question, whether diaplacental transmission of *N. caninum* could be controlled by metaphylactic chemotherapy using toltrazuril (Gottstein et al., 2005). The group could show that toltrazuril can contribute to the control of congenital neosporosis in experimentally infected C57BL/6 mice. Toltrazuril-treatment significantly reduced pre- and perinatal losses. Furthermore, the mother themselves appeared to be protected. Vertical transmission was markedly reduced under toltrazuril treatment, as most of the newborns from treated dams were PCR-negative and had no detectable abnormalities in the brain.

## 4. The immune system of newborn mice

Not much is known about the immune system in foetal as well as newborn mammalians. Most studies concentrate on the immune response within the first days of life.

Some important differences between adults and neonatal responses include: (I) the kinetics of cytokine production and responsiveness to adjuvant during the primary response; and (II) the contribution of spleen and lymph node to secondary responses. The capacity to develop a balanced Th1/Th2 primary effector response is fully mature within the first week of life, but the secondary response is predominated by a Th2 profile (Adkins and Du, 1998). Exposition of newborns to antigens under a variety of conditions showed that murine neonates are clearly competent to develop adult-like Th1 and cytotoxic T-lymphocyte (CTL) functions. Furthermore, the responses were remarkably plastic and highly dependent on the conditions of antigen exposure (Adkins, 2005). The immune status during pregnancy, and particularly the foetal-placental environment producing cytokines (Th2 cytokines, such as IL-4, IL-5 and IL-10), are likely to influence foetuses and subsequently newborns, resulting in a regulation towards Th2 response in early life (Morein et al., 2002). However, this causes an increased susceptibility to intracellular parasites.

An efficient way to vaccinate newborns against intracellular pathogens is of high relevance. A DNA vaccination *in utero* could lead to efficient priming of specific T-cell responses and under appropriate conditions, the foetal immune system could be programmed towards a Th1 response (Rizzi et al., 2005).

## 5. Dendritic cells

Dendritic cells (DCs) are the most potent professional antigen-presenting cells (APCs) that ingest antigens by phagocytosis or pinocytosis. DCs degrade the antigen in lysosomes and display fragments of it on their surface for presentation to T-cell receptors (TCRs). Up-regulation of B7-1 (CD80) and B7-2 (CD86) expression by APCs represents a central event in activation of naïve T-cells to infectious agents (Thompson, 1995). DC1-type dendritic cells secrete IL-12 and stimulate pre-Th cells to mature into Th1 cells. DC-2 dendritic cells stimulate pre-Th cells to mature into Th2 cells. One the other hand, IL-2 and transforming growth factor-β (TGF-β) production by DCs support regulatory T-cell activity and thus an immunosuppressive or immunotolerant pathway (Belkaid and Oldenhove, 2008; Sojka et al., 2008).

DCs exist in different stages of function and maturation. There is a tight correlation between DC maturation and the intracellular antigen-processing pathway, which is important for cross-presentation. Immature DCs reside within non-lymphoid tissues, where they actively capture and process antigen. Contact with pro-inflammatory cytokines and bacterial products induce DC maturation. Upon activation, DCs migrate to secondary lymphoid tissues, where they reside as potent stimulators of naïve T-cells. IL-12 production results in Th1 priming and IL-10 production results in Th2 priming function. Only early immature DCs transported ingested antigens from the endocytic compartments into the cytosol and performed cross-presentation (Hotta et al., 2006). Both mouse classical and plasmacytoid DCs generated from bone marrow as well as DCs generated from lymphoid tissue were able to induce Th1 or Th2 responses. This function was found to depend on the dose of antigen, the state of maturation of DCs and the stimulation of DCs by pathogen-derived products (Boonstra et al., 2003). DCs can directly sense pathogen components via toll-like receptors (TLRs). They responded to this recognition by up-regulation of surface co-stimulatory molecules, secretion of cytokines and chemokines enhancing antigen presentation, and migrating to secondary lymphoid tissues (Iwasaki and Medzhitov, 2004).

Innate lymphocytes – natural killer (NK) cells, natural killer T (NKT) cells and γδT-cells – induce DC maturation, which in turn expands the numbers and function of both innate and adaptive lymphocytes. The interaction of DCs with innate lymphocytes represents a major control mechanism for immunity that is independent of TLR ligands. The consequences of innate lymphocyte interactions with DCs are that: (I) innate cells induce DC maturation through cell contact mechanisms that are still unknown; (II) DCs expand the number and enhance the function of innate lymphocytes; (III) maturing DCs process antigens, particularly from cells lysed by innate lymphocytes, eliciting adaptive Th1 immunity; and (IV) this cross talk seems to occur largely in secondary lymphoid organs (Münz et al., 2005).

Sun et al. (2003) demonstrated that mouse spleen DCs developed right after birth could act as an innate host defence and resistance system to pathogens, but also as competent partners for the stimulation of T-cell-adaptive immunity. Following microbial stimulation, neonatal DCs produced high amounts of IL-12 and IFN-γ. It was found that cytokine-mediated control of IL-12 production was identical for neonatal and adult DCs. The high capacity of neonatal DCs to produce IL-12, IFN-γ and IFN-α showed that DCs could efficiently participate in natural resistance against intracellular pathogens. Furthermore, it was found that neonatal and adult spleen DCs induced comparable allergenic CD8 T-cell stimulation, and that they were also capable of triggering CTL and Th1 responses. Neonatal DCs could be efficiently activated, leading to production of IL-12 (Th1 polarization factor) and to the up-regulation of major histocompatibility complex (MHC) and co-stimulatory molecules (for efficient T-cell priming). Altogether, no developmental immaturity of neonatal DC functions was found (Sun et al., 2003).

## 5.1. DCs and intracellular parasites

TLRs play an important role in the innate recognition of pathogens by DCs. DCs activated by TLR ligands have been shown to induce an early influx and activation of NK cells in the lymph nodes and to be important for the development of Th1 responses. TLR11 was implicated as a receptor for apicomplexan protozoan parasites and for IL-12 production by DCs. One chemically defined ligand for TLR11, the *T. gondii* profilin, generated a potent IL-12 response in murine DCs that was dependent on myeloid differentiation factor 88 (Yarovinsky et al., 2005). *T. gondii* profilin belongs to the class of actin-binding proteins and profilin-like homologs are clearly present in other apicomplexan parasites.

Extracts of *T. gondii* were found to activate DCs and to stimulate IL-12 production by DCs (Reis e Sousa et al., 1997). Full induction of DC functions by this parasite involved both, G-protein-coupled and MyD88-dependent signalling pathways (Scanga et al., 2002). By contrast, active *T. gondii* invasion of immature DCs suppressed the ability of these cells to participate in innate immunity and to induce adaptive immune responses (McKee et al., 2004). Infection of immature DCs allowed parasites to disseminate from the site of infection within cells undergoing steady-state migration to draining lymphoid organs. It was shown that *T. gondii* induced a state of hypermotility in infected DCs *in vitro* and that parasite-infected DCs promoted dissemination of *Toxoplasma in vivo* (Lambert et al., 2006). This benefited that parasites reached the brain and skeletal muscles, where tachyzoites could undergo differentiation into encysted bradyzoite forms to establish chronic infection and ensure parasite transmission.

Mice (BALB/c) infection experiments demonstrated that *N. caninum* stimulated antigen presentation on splenic DCs (Veeraseatakul and Chutipongvivate, 2005). MHC class II glycoproteins and the co-stimulatory ligand CD80 were significantly increased in DCs from *N. caninum*-infected mice. Since the presence of CD80 favoured the activation of Th1 lymphocytes, DCs might play an important role not only in initiating adaptive immunity, but also in early induction of innate immunity. Moreover, up-regulation of MHC class II molecule expression on splenic DCs might be associated with host survival despite parasite infection.

# Summary of publications

1. **NcGRA2 as a molecular target to assess the parasiticidal activity of toltrazuril against *Neospora caninum*. Strohbusch M., Müller N., Hemphill A., Greif G. and Gottstein B. (2008). Parasitology; Aug 135(9); 1065-73**

A molecular assay was established that allows to distinguish between live and dead parasites. Live parasites can be detected by measuring the mRNA level of specific genes, making use of the specific mRNA available in live cells. The *NcGra2* gene of *N. caninum*, which is known to be expressed in both tachyzoites and bradyzoites, was used to establish a RT-PCR, for monitoring parasite viability. Validation of the system *in vitro* was achieved upon *Neospora*-infected cells that were treated with toltrazuril. Quantitative RT-PCR demonstrated that a 10-day-toltrazuril-treatment exerted a parasitostatic activity, whereas a 14-day-treatment was necessary to obtain parasiticidal effects. This assay has a potential to be widely used in the development of novel drugs against *N. caninum*, this in view to distinguish between parasiticidal and parasitostatic efficacy of given compounds.

2. **NcGRA2-RT-PCR to detect live versus dead parasites in *Neospora caninum*-infected mice. Strohbusch M., Müller N., Hemphill A., Greif G. and Gottstein B. (2008). The Open Parasitology Journal; in press**

The NcGRA2-RT-PCR based on RNA was optimized to detect live parasites in tissue from *Neospora caninum*-infected mice and compared with the conventional inoculation of diagnostic specimen into cell culture. C57BL/6 mice were experimentally infected with Nc-1 tachyzoites and subsequently euthanized 6 or 12 days post infection (dpi). Selected organs were used to search for parasites by; (I) PCR using genomic DNA (gDNA); (II) PCR using cDNA; and (III) *in vitro* inoculation of cell culture. At 6 dpi, gDNA was present in almost all organs, whereas live parasites detected with NcGRA2-RT-PCR and parasites growth in cell culture were primarily found in lungs. At 12 dpi, parasite gDNA was mostly present in brains. The viability of these parasites was confirmed both with NcGRA2-RT-PCR and growth of parasites in cell culture. Concluding, the NcGRA2-RT-PCR represents a fast, easy and safe method for viable parasite detection, and therefore is an attractive alternative to the *in vitro* cultivation approach.

3. **Toltrazuril treatment of congenitally acquired *Neospora caninum*-infection in newborn mice.** Strohbusch M., Müller N., Hemphill A., Greif G. and Gottstein B. (manuscript).

Wild-type mice were infected with *N. caninum* tachyzoites during pregnancy, yielding a transplacental infection of developing foetuses. Subsequently, the congenitally infected newborn mice were treated either once or three-times with toltrazuril or a corresponding placebo. These treatments had no negative effect on newborns as non-infected treated pups developed normally. Already one application of toltrazuril was able to delay the outbreak of neosporosis in newborn mice significantly. Toltrazuril treatment resulted in significantly higher survival rates compared to placebo-treated pups. Further, the number of diseased and *Neospora*-positive pups was markedly reduced after three toltrazuril applications compared to all other groups. The three-time-treatment also resulted in the highest antibody response. Treatment with three applications of toltrazuril has the best positive effect for controlling the course of infection in congenitally *N. caninum*-infected newborn mice.

4. **Survival of *Neospora caninum* inside mouse bone marrow-derived dendritic cells and induction of cytokine expression.** Strohbusch M., Müller N., Hemphill A., Margos M., Grandgirard D., Greif G. and Gottstein B. (manuscript).

So far, nothing is known about the invasion and survival ability of *Neospora caninum* in mouse bone marrow-derived dendritic cells (mBMDCs), as well as cytokine expression pattern after DCs had contact with tachyzoites. In the present study, we stimulated mBMDCs with viable (untreated) and different kinds of inactivated parasites and determined invasion and survival ability by NcGRA2-RT-PCR and transmission electron microscopy, and cytokine expression by RT-PCR and cytokine-ELISA. Untreated *N. caninum* tachyzoites were able to invade, survive and proliferate within DCs. Inactivated parasites were phagocytosed by DCs and non-viablity was proven with NcGRA2-RT-PCR. Cytokine expression analysis exhibited that both, viable and inactivated parasites, stimulate DCs in a way that they express IL-12p40, IL-10 and TNF-α, whereas IL-4 levels were below detection limit. The work present here, was a first approach to determine survival and proliferation ability of *N. caninum* within mBMDCs and cytokine expression pattern of DCs after stimulation with parasites.

**Accepted publication**

# *NcGRA2* as a molecular target to assess the parasiticidal activity of toltrazuril against *Neospora caninum*

M. STROHBUSCH[1], N. MÜLLER[1], A. HEMPHILL[1], G. GREIF[2] and B. GOTTSTEIN[1*]

[1] *Institute of Parasitology, University of Berne, Laenggass-Strasse 122, CH-3012 Berne, Switzerland*
[2] *Bayer HealthCare AG, Leverkusen, Germany*

(*Received 19 December 2007; revised 27 February and 23 April 2008; accepted 28 April 2008; first published online 13 June 2008*)

### SUMMARY

The treatment of *Neospora caninum* infection in the bovine host is still at an experimental stage. In contrast to the *in vivo* situation, a wide range of compounds have been intensively investigated in cell-culture-based assays. Tools to demonstrate efficacy of treatment have remained conventional including morphological and cell biological criteria. In this work, we present a molecular assay that allows the distinction between live and dead parasites. Live parasites can be detected by measuring the mRNA level of specific genes, making use of the specific mRNA available in live cells. The *NcGra2* gene of *N. caninum*, which is known to be expressed in both tachyzoites and bradyzoites, was used to establish a quantitative real-time RT-PCR, for monitoring parasite viability. Validation of the system *in vitro* was achieved using *Neospora*-infected cells that had been treated for 2–20 days with 30 µg/ml toltrazuril. *NcGRA2*-RT-real time PCR demonstrated that a 10-day toltrazuril-treatment exerted parasitostatic activity, as assessed by the presence of *NcGRA2*-transcripts, whereas after a 14-day treatment period no *NcGRA2*-transcripts were detected, showing that the parasites were no longer viable. Concurrently, extended culture for a period of 4 weeks in the absence of the drug following the 14-day toltrazuril treatment did not lead to further parasite proliferation, confirming the parasiticidal effect of the treatment. This assay has the potential to be widely used in the development of novel drugs against *N. caninum*, with a view to distinguishing between parasiticidal and parasitostatic efficacy of given compounds.

Key words: *Neospora caninum*, RT-PCR, cell-culture assay, toltrazuril.

### INTRODUCTION

The main problem associated with the apicomplexan parasite *Neospora caninum* and the corresponding disease, neosporosis, is abortion in cattle (Dubey, 2003), which represents a serious veterinary health and economic problem within livestock production (Hemphill and Gottstein, 2000; Dubey *et al.* 2007).

So far, efficacy of experimental treatment and vaccination *in vitro* or *in vivo* has been determined upon use of morphological criteria of affected parasites (microscopy or TEM), differential demonstration of the absence or presence of parasite-induced lesions upon (immuno-) histology, and PCR-based detection of parasite DNA in such lesions and affected organs (Kritzner *et al.* 2002; Darius *et al.* 2004*b*; Esposito *et al.* 2005). However, the presence of parasite DNA or antigens in infected tissue does not necessarily provide information on parasite viability, and conventional *in vivo/in vitro* tests are being used by inoculating appropriate samples into mice or cell cultures (Dubey *et al.* 2007). Since these methods can often be time-consuming and inconclusive, we tackled the problem by addressing parasite mRNA as a target to demonstrate viability or non-viability of organisms. Although the genome of *N. caninum* is not yet fully described, several genes could be identified by comparison with the related parasite *Toxoplasma gondii*. Immunoscreening of a cDNA library derived from mRNA of *N. caninum* tachyzoites resulted in the identification of a clone with a deduced protein sequence exhibiting a significant homology of the gene product to the 28 kDa (GRA2) antigen of *T. gondii* (Ellis *et al.* 2000). In *T. gondii* the *TgGra2* gene product is an excreted-secreted antigen, which is stored in the dense granules and secreted in the parasitophorous vacuole after host cell invasion (Mercier *et al.* 1993). Since the corresponding mRNA was abundantly present in *N. caninum* tachyzoites, it was assumed that the gene is highly expressed in this stage (Ellis *et al.* 2000). The *TgGra2* gene of *T. gondii* was found to be constitutively expressed in both, tachyzoites and bradyzoites (Manger *et al.* 1998). In *N. caninum* the NcGRA2 protein was found to be associated with the parasitophorous tubular network in tachyzoites and incorporated into the cyst wall of *in vitro* derived bradyzoites (Vonlaufen *et al.* 2004).

The need for the development of effective pro- or metaphylactic measures against bovine neosporosis has been widely addressed and discussed (Kritzner

* Corresponding author: Institute of Parasitology, Vetsuisse Faculty, University of Bern, Laenggass-Strasse 122, CH-3001 Bern, Switzerland. Tel: +41 31 631 24 18. E-mail: bruno.gottstein@ipa.unibe.ch

et al. 2002; Gottstein et al. 2001; Innes et al. 2002; Häsler et al. 2006 a, b). Chemotherapy is being discussed as an interesting alternative to the vaccination strategy (Häsler et al. 2006 a, b). Toltrazuril, a symmetric triazinone derivative, was shown to exhibit anti-coccidial activity against cyst-forming and non-cyst-forming coccidians (Haberkorn, 1996). The effects of toltrazuril on the fine structure and multiplication of N. caninum were studied in cell culture employing light and electron microscopy (Darius et al. 2004 b). The authors demonstrated considerable damage, induced in N. caninum tachyzoites that were incubated in 30 $\mu$g/ml toltrazuril for periods of up to 12 h, and they concluded that the drug was exhibiting parasiticidal activity. In the murine model of experimental N. caninum infection, toltrazuril treatment prevented severe clinical signs and the formation of cerebral lesions (Gottstein et al. 2001; Darius et al. 2004 a). However, Ammann et al. (2004) clearly demonstrated that an efficient metaphylaxis requires at least a T-cell-mediated immunological support in mice. We now used NcGra2 as a target gene to demonstrate viability or non-viability of N. caninum in affected host cells following treatment with the anti-parasitic compound toltrazuril.

MATERIALS AND METHODS

Tissue-culture media, biochemicals and drugs

If not otherwise stated, all tissue-culture media were purchased from Gibco-BRL (Basel, Switzerland) and biochemical reagents were from Sigma (St Louis, MO). Toltrazuril formulated for tissue culture was provided by Dr Gisela Greif (Bayer HealthCare AG, Germany), stock solutions at 30 mg/ml were prepared in dimethyl sulfoxide (DMSO) and stored at 4 °C for not longer than 1 month.

Tissue culture and parasite purification

Cultures of Vero cells were maintained in RPMI 1640 medium (Gibco-BRL) supplemented with 5% fetal calf serum (FCS), 4 mM L-glutamine and 100 U/ml penicillin G, 100 $\mu$g/ml streptomycin and 0.25 $\mu$g/ml amphotericin B at 37 °C with 5% $CO_2$. Cultures were trypsinized at least once a week. Human foreskin fibroblasts (HFF) were maintained in Dulbecco's modified Eagle's medium (DMEM) containing the same additives and were identically treated. N. caninum (Nc-1 and Nc-Liverpool isolates) and T. gondii (RH isolate) tachyzoites were maintained in Vero cell monolayer cultures, during which time FCS was replaced with immunoglobulin G-free horse serum. Tachyzoites were harvested when they were still intracellular by trypsinization of infected Vero cells followed by repeated passage through a 25-gauge needle. Host cell debris was removed from the parasites by separation on Sephadex-G25 columns as previously described (Hemphill et al. 1996). The tachyzoites were counted using a Neubauer chamber and cell pellets were frozen at $-80$ °C prior to DNA and RNA extraction to develop and examine the sensitivity and specificity of the PCR. Furthermore, freshly isolated and counted parasites were diluted for in vitro drug treatment assays.

Host cell infection and in vitro drug treatment assays

HFF were grown to confluent monolayer in 24-well tissue-culture plates and infected with $5 \times 10^4$ purified Nc-1 tachyzoites per well for 2 h at 37 °C with 5% $CO_2$, as previously described (Esposito et al. 2005). Unbound parasites were removed by washing in DMEM, and infected monolayers were maintained in supplemented DMEM containing the indicated drug concentration (see below). Controls contained the appropriate amounts of the solvent DMSO alone. The cultures were maintained under treatment at 37 °C with 5% $CO_2$ for various periods of time and checked daily by light microscopy. DMSO- or drug-containing medium was changed every day. A control experiment was done to specifically assess the effect of the solvent DMSO alone on the parasite proliferation and survival in infected HFF monolayers. Infected monolayers were maintained under DMSO treatment in the absence of DMSO for 20 days. DMSO was used in a 1:1000 dilution, corresponding to the DMSO concentration in drug-containing medium. Samples for monitoring parasites were collected (as indicated below) on days 0, 3, 5, 7, 11 and 20, following initiation of the treatment. In experimental part 1, different concentrations of toltrazuril were tested. Infected monolayers were maintained in medium containing 30, 60 or 90 $\mu$g/ml toltrazuril for 2 days. Samples were collected as indicated below. In experimental part 2, the short-term effect of toltrazuril on infected monolayers was assessed. Therefore, infected monolayers were treated with 30 $\mu$g/ml toltrazuril or a corresponding amount of DMSO solvent for 2 days. Samples for monitoring parasite survival by RT-PCR were taken at day 0, 1 and 2, following initiation of the treatment. Experimental part 3 investigated the long-term effect of toltrazuril and the putative recurrence of the proliferative activity of the treated parasites. For this, infected monolayers were treated with 30 $\mu$g/ml toltrazuril for 3-20 days. The follow-up analyses of DMSO-treated control cultures were stopped after 6 days, as the control experiment did not show a negative effect of DMSO (Fig. 2). Samples for monitoring parasite survival by RT-PCR were taken at days 3, 10, 14 and 20, following initiation of drug treatment. Furthermore, infected monolayers were trypsinized at day 3, 10 and 14 and washed in DMEM. After centrifugation, the pellet was resuspended in 4 volumes of supplemented DMEM, added to 4 wells with fresh HFF monolayers and maintained for up to 32 days in the absence of the drug.

Experimental part 4 was designed to assess the effect of toltrazuril on an established *in vitro* infection. For this, HFF monolayers were infected and parasites were subsequently allowed to proliferate in the absence of the drug. After 3 days, 30 μg/ml toltrazuril was added and the cultures were maintained for another 4 days under treatment.

For sample collection, the medium was removed and wells were washed with PBS. The cellular material was taken up in 400 μl of RTL$^+$ buffer (AllPrep DNA/RNA kit; QIAGEN, Basel, Switzerland) containing 1% β-mercaptoethanol, then transferred to Eppendorf tubes and frozen at −80 °C prior to DNA and RNA extraction. Each assay in a given experiment was carried out in triplicate.

### DNA/RNA extraction and cDNA synthesis

DNA and RNA purification were performed using the AllPrep DNA/RNA kit (QIAGEN) according to the standard protocol suitable for cell cultures. Frozen cell pellets were lysed in 750 μl of RTL$^+$ buffer containing 1% β-mercaptoethanol. Frozen lysates were allowed to thaw at 37 °C. All purification steps were performed at room temperature. DNA was eluted in 60 μl of AE buffer and RNA in 60 μl of RNAse-free water. DNA was boiled at 95 °C for 3 min and frozen at −80 °C prior to PCR. RNA was boiled at 95 °C for 3 min and immediately used for cDNA synthesis.

### Reverse Transcription

cDNA synthesis was performed using the Omniscript® Reverse Transcription kit (QIAGEN) according to the standard protocol for first-strand cDNA synthesis. Briefly, 0.5 μg random Primer (Promega, Wallisellen, Switzerland) and 2 μl of RNA were used in a final volume of 20 μl reaction mix and incubated for 1 h at 37 °C. cDNA was boiled at 95 °C for 3 min and frozen at −80 °C prior to PCR.

### Conventional PCR

Detection of parasite-specific DNA by Nc5-PCR was done as previously described (Müller *et al.* 1996) with *N. caninum*-specific primers Np21plus and Np6plus in a thermal cycler (Gene Amp PCR System model 9700; Applied Biosystems, Basel Switzerland). For the mix, 20 pmol of each primer and 1 μl of DNA in a final volume of 25 μl were used.

For detection of parasite-specific cDNA, the forward primer NcGRA2-F1 (5′GATGATGTTAGAGAATCAATGGC 3′) and the reverse primer NcGRA2-R2 (5′CCGTCCTTCTCCATCGTCC 3′) were designed using nucleotide sequence data available from the GenBank databases (http://www.ncbi.nlm.nih.gov/GenBank/index.html) under the Accession number AF196293. PCR was performed using 25 pmol of each primer and 1 μl of cDNA in a final volume of 25 μl in a thermal cycler for 40 cycles (94 °C, 30 sec; 60 °C, 30 sec; 72 °C, 2 min), followed by a final primer extension at 72 °C for 15 min. The PCR amplified a product of 486 bp of the *NcGra2* gene (Fig. 1A).

Both PCR-mixes were performed using the AmpliTaq® DNA polymerase kit (Applied Biosystems). To prevent carry-over contamination from previous reactions, the samples were incubated with uracyl DNA glycosylase (UDG; Roche Diagnostics, Basel, Switzerland) for 10 min at 20 °C. The UDG was inactivated by incubation at 95 °C for 2 min. Each run included a negative (water) and a positive (purified parasites) sample.

### Quantitative real-time PCR

Quantitative real-time Nc5-PCR based on DNA was performed on the LightCycler instrument (Roche Diagnostics) as previously described (Müller *et al.* 2002) using *N. caninum*-specific primers Np21plus and Np6plus, Nc5-specific hybridization probes 3FL and 5CL and 1:410 diluted DNA.

Quantitative real-time RT-PCR based on cDNA was performed using the QuantiTec™SYBR® Green PCR kit (QIAGEN), gene-specific primers NcGRA2-F1 and -R2 and 1:41 diluted cDNA. After activation of the DNA polymerase for 15 min at 95 °C, PCR was performed for 50 cycles (94 °C, 15 sec; 58 °C, 15 sec; 72 °C, 30 sec) with a single acquisition mode at 85 °C, followed by a melting curve. Both PCRs were performed with 4.1 μl of sample in a final volume of 10 μl. To avoid carry-over contamination, UDG was added to the mix. As external standards, samples containing DNA or cDNA equivalents from 100, 10 and 1 *N. caninum* tachyzoite(s) were included. Parasite number was calculated by assessing mean values (plus standard deviations) from triplicate determinations.

Quantitative real-time RT-PCR for the amplification of host cell α-actin was performed using the QuantiTec™SYBR®Green PCR kit (QIAGEN) as described previously (Müller *et al.* 2003). The PCR included forward primer α-ac1, reverse primer α-ac2 and 4 μl of 1:10 diluted cDNA in a 10 μl standard reaction.

### Statistical analysis

For time-course experiments, the significance of the differences between end-point values of the control and experimental assays was determined by Student's *t* test, using the Microsoft Excel program.

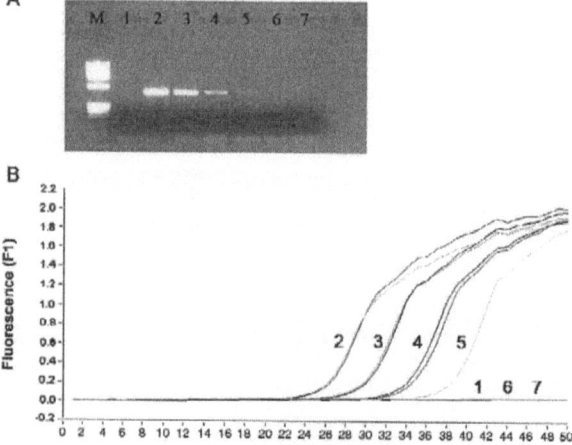

Fig. 1. NcGRA2-RT-PCR sensitivity. cDNA was diluted and conventional PCR (A) and real-time RT-PCR (B) was performed using the *NcGRA2*-specific primers. Dilutions included 100 (2), 10 (3), 1 (4), 0.1 (5), 0.01 (6) or 0.001 (7) parasite equivalents. For the real-time RT-PCR every dilution was performed in duplicate. Using cDNA, the PCR amplified a product of 468 bp. M: DNA-marker $\Phi$X174; 1: negative control.

$P$ values of $<0.05$ were considered statistically significant.

RESULTS

*Sensitivity and specificity of PCR*

The nucleotide sequence of the *NcGRA2* gene was derived from the GenBank database under Accession number AF196293. A primer pair was designed that included the exon/exon fusion side of the gene. The product amplified by conventional PCR using cDNA had a size of 468 bp (Fig. 1A). To assess the sensitivity of the RT-PCR, cDNA samples from purified Nc-1 tachyzoites were run at different dilutions (Fig. 1A). Visualization of the PCR products showed an end-point sensitivity of 0.1 parasite equivalents per PCR reaction. The PCR was specific for cDNA as there was no detectable product after the amplification of the same amount of parasite DNA (data not shown). For quantification of the number of parasites in a given sample, the conventional RT-PCR was transformed into a real-time RT-PCR. The sensitivity of the real-time RT-PCR was determined with cDNA samples from purified Nc-1 tachyzoites at different dilutions (Fig. 1B). The real-time RT-PCR showed an end-point sensitivity of 0.1 parasite equivalents per PCR reaction. To test the species specificity, conventional RT-PCR was carried out with NcLiv tachyzoites and *Toxoplasma* RH tachyzoites. The PCR was positive for *Neospora* tachyzoites but negative for *Toxoplasma* tachyzoites (data not shown).

*In vitro treatment with toltrazuril*

The NcGRA2-RT-PCR-assay was used to assess the efficacy of toltrazuril *in vitro*. As toltrazuril was dissolved in DMSO, a control experiment was carried out to determine the effect of the solvent DMSO on parasite proliferation and survival. DMSO had no negative effect on parasite survival, as quantitative real-time RT-PCR detected similar amounts of parasites in the DMSO-treated and -untreated cultures after 20 days (Fig. 2). Due to the fact, that the tachyzoites egressed and destroyed most of the host cell monolayer, a decrease of parasites was observed from day 5 onwards in both, DMSO-treated and -untreated cultures.

Different concentrations of toltrazuril were tested on infected HFF host cells *in vitro*. Cultures were grown in medium containing 30, 60 or 90 $\mu$g/ml toltrazuril for 2 days. Quantitative real-time RT-PCR revealed no difference in the parasite amount between the 3 used concentrations (data not shown). Therefore, all further experiments were done with a toltrazuril concentration of 30 $\mu$g/ml. To assess the short-term effect of toltrazuril, infected cell cultures were grown in drug-containing medium for 2 days. A significant difference in the parasite number was first observed after 2 days of treatment when compared with the untreated culture (Fig. 3).

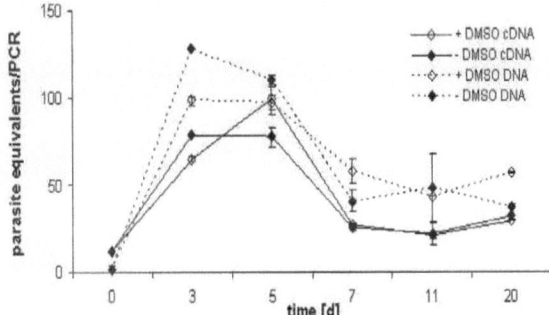

Fig. 2. Effect of the solvent DMSO on parasite proliferation and survival. HFF monolayers were infected with *Neosporum caninum* tachyzoites, and at 2 h p.i. DMSO (1:1000) was added. The control cultures contained medium without DMSO. Treatment was stopped at 3, 5, 7, 11 and 20 days p.i. The y-axis shows the number of parasite equivalents per quantitative real-time NcGRA2-RT-PCR (detection of *Neospora* cDNA; filled line) and quantitative real-time Nc5-PCR (detection of *Neospora* genomic DNA; dotted line). The amount of parasites decreased from day 5 on, due to the lysis of the host cells.

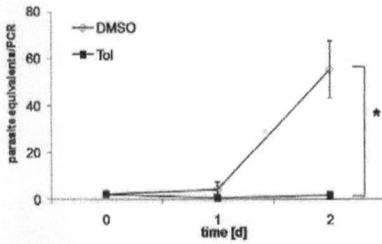

Fig. 3. Short-term effect of toltrazuril. HFF monolayers were infected with *Neospora caninum* tachyzoites, and at 2 h p.i. 30 µg/ml toltrazuril (Tol) was added. Samples were collected at day 0 and days 1 and 2 p.i. The y-axis shows the number of parasite equivalents per quantitative real-time NcGRA2-RT-PCR. There is a significantly lower amount of parasites at 2 days p.i. in the toltrazuril-treated sample compared to the DMSO control (* $P < 0.05$).

Longer-term treatment assays were carried out to determine the treatment duration necessary for parasiticidal activity (Fig. 4). Quantitative real-time NcGRA2-RT-PCR was unable to detect any parasites after a 14-day-treatment period (Fig. 4A). A comparison of the parasite numbers, calculated by means of DNA and cDNA, revealed that DNA is still detectable after 14 days of drug treatment, while no NcGRA2-RNA is being produced anymore at this time-point, indicating that the tachyzoites detected by real-time PCR were non-viable (Fig. 4B). In order to verify this, the infected and drug-treated cultures were maintained after the treatment in drug-free medium for up to 4 weeks (Fig. 4C). *Neospora*

was able to restart proliferation even after 10 days of exposure to toltrazuril. However, no recurrence of the parasite in cell culture was observed after the treatment period of 14 days. Furthermore, quantitative real-time PCR, based on DNA and cDNA, did not detect any parasites in the culture samples. Host cells were not negatively affected by the treatment, as microscopical observation showed no morphological alterations to indicate destruction. Further, the host cell α-actin transcription level, detected by quantitative real-time RT-PCR, remained constant over the treatment period (data not shown).

Toltrazuril also acts against an established *in vitro* infection of host cells with *Neospora*. Cultures were infected and grown for 3 days in the absence of the drug. Addition of toltrazuril, after establishment of the infection *in vitro*, reduced the parasite number (Fig. 5).

DISCUSSION

The apicomplexan parasite *Neospora caninum* is an obligate intracellular parasite, infection of which is associated with abortion in cattle. To date, there is no effective treatment for cattle available (Andrianarivo *et al.* 2000; Innes and Vermeulen, 2006) but a considerable number of potentially useful compounds were tested in cell-culture-based assays (Lindsay and Dubey, 1989; Lindsay *et al.* 1994). In most cases, the effects of a given compound were microscopically examined (Darius *et al.* 2004b), or parasite numbers were determined either by microscopical counting of the parasites or by extraction of DNA and quantitative real-time PCR (Esposito *et al.* 2005). However, while these techniques provided information on the proliferation inhibitory effects of a given compound,

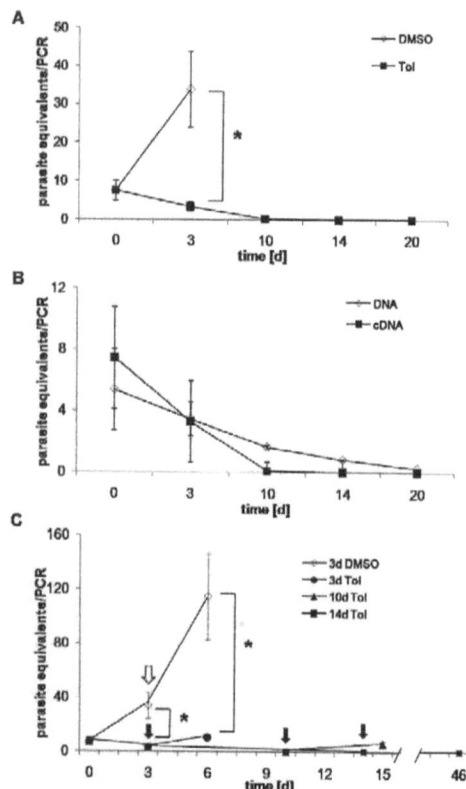

Fig. 4. Long-term effect of toltrazuril and re-start of parasite proliferation. HFF monolayers were infected with *Neospora caninum* tachyzoites, and at 2 h p.i. 30 μg/ml toltrazuril (Tol) was added. (A) Treatment was stopped at 3, 10, 14 and 20 days p.i. The y-axis shows the number of parasite equivalents per quantitative real-time NcGRA2-RT-PCR. As assessed by NcGRA2-RT-PCR, there was no detectable parasite in the sample after 14 and 20 days of treatment. (B) Comparison of parasite numbers, as detected by quantitative real-time Nc5-PCR (detection of *Neospora* genomic DNA) and quantitative real-time NcGRA2-RT-PCR (detection of *Neospora* cDNA). Note that there is still genomic DNA but no detectable cDNA in the 14-day treated sample. (C) After the indicated treatment duration, cultures were maintained without DMSO (after 3 days, open arrow) or toltrazuril (after 3, 10 and 14 days, closed arrows) for up to 4 weeks. Note that no restart of proliferation was observed after 14 days of treatment. There is a significantly lower amount of parasites in the toltrazuril-treated samples compared to the DMSO control at days 3 and 6 p.i. (* $P<0.05$).

they did not allow distinction between live and dead parasites following a given treatment. The aim of the present study was to develop a method that could be used to distinguish between live and dead *N. caninum* parasites. To validate the method, *Neospora* tachyzoites were treated *in vitro* with toltrazuril, a drug that was shown earlier to exhibit considerable anti-parasitic activity against *N. caninum* (Gottstein *et al.* 2001; Darius *et al.* 2004 a, b).

To detect only the live parasites, we developed a PCR using cDNA based on mRNA of the *NcGRA2* gene, making use of the specific mRNA of an antigen that is expressed in both tachyzoite and bradyzoite stages. The *NcGRA2* gene sequence contains 2 exons and 1 intron and is highly expressed in tachyzoites (Ellis *et al.* 2000). The dense granule protein NcGRA2 was also detected in *in vitro*-derived bradyzoites (Vonlaufen *et al.* 2004). The

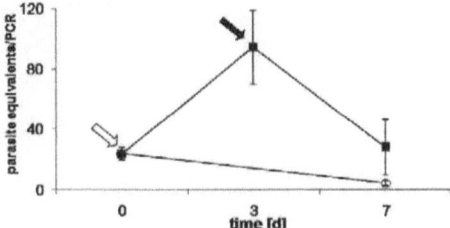

Fig. 5. Effect of toltrazuril on an established *Neospora caninum* infection. Infected fibroblasts were grown for 3 days without toltrazuril to establish an infection. Treatment started 0 (open arrow) or 3 (closed arrow) days p.i. Note that toltrazuril treatment reduced the number of parasites after an established infection, as assessed by quantitative real-time NcGRA2-RT-PCR.

NcGRA2-RT-PCR developed herein was specific for cDNA derived from *N. caninum* Nc-1 and Nc-Liverpool strain tachyzoites. As the NcGRA2-specific primers included the exon/exon fusion site, the NcGRA2 DNA sequence was not amplified in this reaction. Despite a 56% similarity between the *Neospora* and the *Toxoplasma GRA2* sequences (Ellis et al. 2000), the NcGRA2-RT-PCR was highly specific for the NcGRA2 sequence. These observations indicated that the new NcGRA2-RT-PCR should be considered as a useful tool to detect live *Neospora* parasites, especially due to its high sensitivity of 0·1 parasite equivalents per reaction.

To validate the NcGRA2-RT-PCR, *in vitro* treatment of *N. caninum* with toltrazuril was performed. The solvent DMSO itself has no negative effect on parasite survival. Similar amounts of parasites were found in DMSO-treated and -untreated cultures after a time-period of 20 days. Previous studies had already indicated that toltrazuril exhibits profound anti-parasitic activity, inducing considerable damage in *N. caninum* tachyzoites upon *in vitro* treatment and limiting parasite proliferation and dissemination in experimentally infected mice and cattle (Gottstein et al. 2001, 2005; Kritzner et al. 2002; Darius et al. 2004a,b; Haerdi et al. 2006). After microscopical examination of *in vitro* toltrazuril (30 μg/ml)-treated parasites, Darius et al. (2004b) observed severe destruction that was proposed to be lethal. In the cell-culture assay presented in this work, the treatment with 30 μg/ml toltrazuril revealed a significant reduction in the number of parasites after 2 days in treated cultures when compared to untreated cultures. Nevertheless, the 2-day-treated cultures contained viable parasites, as shown by the detection of NcGRA2 mRNA. This is confirmed by the fact that parasites treated for a few days were able to infect new host cells and started proliferation again in the absence of toltrazuril. Thus, when applied for a few days under these experimental conditions, toltrazuril exhibits only parasitostatic activity. In experimentally infected mice a 6-day toltrazuril treatment also had a more parasitostatic rather than a parasiticidal effect (Ammann et al. 2004). A clear parasiticidal effect of toltrazuril, defined in our assay by the failure to detect *NcGRA2* mRNA, was first observed after a continuous long-term treatment of 14 days. However, *N. caninum* DNA was still detectable in the 14-day-treated samples, but the parasites were not viable anymore since they were not able to restart proliferation following drug treatment. Toltrazuril acts specifically against the parasites, as the number of host cells was not affected after the long-term treatment.

In naturally infected animals, usually an established infection has to be treated. In our culture-based assay presented here, toltrazuril could markedly reduce the number of parasites after a 3-day established infection.

In conclusion, we present a novel assay that allows distinction between live and dead *N. caninum* in cell culture. This assay is applicable, for example, in efficacy testing of chemotherapeutically interesting compounds, and was validated with respect to the *in vitro* efficacy of toltrazuril, a drug that is currently being experimentally assessed for the potential treatment of neosporosis in cattle. The fact, that at least 14 days of *in vitro* treatment is necessary to obtain parasiticidal activity of toltrazuril, has important implications for the development of novel treatment strategies for neosporosis in cattle. Further investigations will focus on optimizing this RT-PCR for the detection of live parasites in the tissues of infected animals. Furthermore, we would also like to address the question of whether other stages of the parasite, such as bradyzoites, can be affected by medication, and if the *NcGRA2* mRNA approach can also be used to determine the viability status of fully mature *N. caninum* tissue cysts.

The study was supported by Bayer HealthCare AG (Leverkusen), the Swiss Federal Office of Science and Education (BBW C01.0122 in the frame of COST 854), and the Swiss National Science Foundation (Grant No. 3100A0-112532).

REFERENCES

Ammann, P., Waldvogel, A., Breyer, I., Esposito, M., Müller, N. and Gottstein, B. (2004). The role of B- and T-cell immunity in toltrazuril-treated C57BL/6 WT, microMT and nude mice experimentally infected with *Neospora caninum*. *Parasitology Research* 93, 178–187.

Andrianarivo, A. G., Rowe, J. D., Barr, B. C., Anderson, M. L., Packham, A. E., Sverlow, K. W., Choromanski, L., Loui, C., Grace, A. and Conrad, P. A. (2000). A POLYGEN-adjuvanted killed *Neospora caninum* tachyzoite preparation failed to prevent foetal infection in pregnant cattle following i.v./i.m. experimental tachyzoite challenge. *International Journal for Parasitology* 30, 985–990.

Darius, A. K., Mehlhorn, H. and Heydorn, A. O. (2004a). Effects of toltrazuril and ponazuril on *Hammondia heydorni* (syn. *Neospora caninum*) infections in mice. *Parasitology Research* 92, 520–522.

Darius, A. K., Mehlhorn, H. and Heydorn, A. O. (2004b). Effects of toltrazuril and ponazuril on the fine structure and multiplication of tachyzoites of the NC-1 strain of *Neospora caninum* (a synonym of *Hammondia heydorni*) in cell cultures. *Parasitology Research* 92, 453–458.

Dubey, J. P. (2003). Review of *Neospora caninum* and neosporosis in animals. *Korean Journal for Parasitology* 41, 1–16.

Dubey, J. P., Schares, G. and Ortega-Mora, L. M. (2007). Epidemiology and control of neosporosis and *Neospora caninum*. *Clinical Microbiology Reviews* 20, 323–367.

Ellis, J. T., Ryce, C., Atkinson, R., Balu, S., Jones, P. and Harper, P. A. (2000). Isolation, characterization and expression of a GRA2 homologue from *Neospora caninum*. *Parasitology* 120, 383–390.

Esposito, M., Stettler, R., Moores, S. L., Pidathala, C., Müller, N., Stachulski, A., Berry, N. G., Rossignol, J. F. and Hemphill, A. (2005). In vitro efficacies of nitazoxanide and other thiazolides against *Neospora caninum* tachyzoites reveal antiparasitic activity independent of the nitro group. *Antimicrobial Agents and Chemotherapy* 49, 3715–3723.

Gottstein, B., Eperon, S., Dai, W. J., Cannas, A., Hemphill, A. and Greif, G. (2001). Efficacy of toltrazuril and ponazuril against experimental *Neospora caninum* infection in mice. *Parasitology Research* 87, 43–48.

Gottstein, B., Razmi, G. R., Ammann, P., Sager, H. and Müller, N. (2005). Toltrazuril treatment to control diaplacental *Neospora caninum* transmission in experimentally infected pregnant mice. *Parasitology* 130, 41–48.

Haberkorn, A. (1996). Chemotherapy of human and animal coccidioses: state and perspectives. *Parasitology Research* 82, 193–199.

Haerdi, C., Haessig, M., Sager, H., Greif, G., Staubli, D. and Gottstein, B. (2006). Humoral immune reaction of newborn calves congenitally infected with *Neospora caninum* and experimentally treated with toltrazuril. *Parasitology Research* 99, 534–540.

Häsler, B., Regula, G., Stark, K. D., Sager, H., Gottstein, B. and Reist, M. (2006a). Financial analysis of various strategies for the control of *Neospora caninum* in dairy cattle in Switzerland. *Preventive Veterinary Medicine* 77, 230–253.

Häsler, B., Stark, K. D., Sager, H., Gottstein, B. and Reist, M. (2006b). Simulating the impact of four control strategies on the population dynamics of *Neospora caninum* infection in Swiss dairy cattle. *Preventive Veterinary Medicine* 77, 254–283.

Hemphill, A. and Gottstein, B. (2000). A European perspective on *Neospora caninum*. *International Journal for Parasitology* 30, 877–924.

Hemphill, A., Gottstein, B. and Kaufmann, H. (1996). Adhesion and invasion of bovine endothelial cells by *Neospora caninum*. *Parasitology* 112, 183–197.

Innes, E. A., Andrianarivo, A. G., Bjorkman, C., Williams, D. J. and Conrad, P. A. (2002). Immune responses to *Neospora caninum* and prospects for vaccination. *Trends in Parasitology* 18, 497–504.

Innes, E. A. and Vermeulen, A. N. (2006). Vaccination as a control strategy against the coccidial parasites *Eimeria*, *Toxoplasma* and *Neospora*. *Parasitology* 133 (Suppl.), S145–S168.

Kritzner, S., Sager, H., Blum, J., Krebber, R., Greif, G. and Gottstein, B. (2002). An explorative study to assess the efficacy of toltrazuril-sulfone (ponazuril) in calves experimentally infected with *Neospora caninum*. *Annals of Clinical Microbiology and Antimicrobials* 1, 4.

Lindsay, D. S. and Dubey, J. P. (1989). Evaluation of anti-coccidial drugs' inhibition of *Neospora caninum* development in cell cultures. *Journal for Parasitology* 75, 990–992.

Lindsay, D. S., Rippey, N. S., Cole, R. A., Parsons, L. C., Dubey, J. P., Tidwell, R. R. and Blagburn, B. L. (1994). Examination of the activities of 43 chemotherapeutic agents against *Neospora caninum* tachyzoites in cultured cells. *American Journal of Veterinary Research* 55, 976–981.

Manger, I. D., Hehl, A., Parmley, S., Sibley, L. D., Marra, M., Hillier, L., Waterston, R. and Boothroyd, J. C. (1998). Expressed sequence tag analysis of the bradyzoite stage of *Toxoplasma gondii*: identification of developmentally regulated genes. *Infection and Immunity* 66, 1632–1637.

Mercier, C., Lecordier, L., Darcy, F., Deslee, D., Murray, A., Tourvieille, B., Maes, P., Capron, A. and Cesbron-Delauw, M. F. (1993). Molecular characterization of a dense granule antigen (Gra 2) associated with the network of the parasitophorous vacuole in *Toxoplasma gondii*. *Molecular and Biochemical Parasitology* 58, 71–82.

Müller, N., Vonlaufen, N., Gianinazzi, C., Leib, S. L. and Hemphill, A. (2002). Application of real-time fluorescent PCR for quantitative assessment of *Neospora caninum* infections in organotypic slice cultures of rat central nervous system tissue. *Journal of Clinical Microbiology* 40, 252–255.

Müller, N., Zimmermann, V., Forster, U., Bienz, M., Gottstein, B. and Welle, M. (2003). PCR-based detection of canine *Leishmania* infections in formalin-fixed and paraffin-embedded skin biopsies: elaboration of a protocol for quality assessment of the diagnostic amplification reaction. *Veterinary Parasitology* **114**, 223–229.

**Müller, N., Zimmermann, V., Hentrich, B. and Gottstein, B.** (1996). Diagnosis of *Neospora caninum* and *Toxoplasma gondii* infection by PCR and DNA hybridization immunoassay. *Journal of Clinical Microbiology* **34**, 2850–2852.

**Vonlaufen, N., Guetg, N., Naguleswaran, A., Müller, N., Bjorkman, C., Schares, G., Von Blumroeder, D., Ellis, J. and Hemphill, A.** (2004). *In vitro* induction of *Neospora caninum* bradyzoites in vero cells reveals differential antigen expression, localization, and host-cell recognition of tachyzoites and bradyzoites. *Infection and Immunity* **72**, 576–583.

**NcGRA2-RT-PCR to detect live versus dead parasites in *Neospora caninum*-infected mice**

Maria Strohbusch[1], Norbert Müller[1], Andrew Hemphill[1], Gisela Greif[2], Bruno Gottstein[1]*

[1]Institute of Parasitology, University of Bern, Laenggass-Strasse 122, CH-3012 Bern, Switzerland
[2]Bayer HealthCare AG, Leverkusen, Germany

*address for correspondence:

Institute of Parasitology
Vetsuisse Faculty
University of Bern
Laenggassstrasse 122
CH-3001 Bern, Switzerland
+41 31 631 24 18
bruno.gottstein@ipa.unibe.ch

Running header: NcGRA2-RT-PCR for live *Neospora caninum*

## Abstract

In the present work, we optimized a recently established NcGRA2-RT-PCR based on RNA to detect live *Neospora caninum* parasites in tissue, and compared the results with the conventional inoculation of diagnostic specimen onto cell culture. C57BL/6 mice were experimentally infected with Nc-1 tachyzoites and subsequently euthanized 6 or 12 days post infection (dpi). Selected organs were used to search for parasites by (i) PCR using genomic DNA (gDNA), (ii) PCR using cDNA and (iii) *in vitro* inoculation of cell culture. At 6 dpi, *Neospora*-gDNA was detected in 34 out of 36 organs. Viable parasites were detected in 11 (NcGRA2-RT-PCR) and 15 (*in vitro* cultivation) out of 36 organs. Comparison of NcGRA2-RT-PCR and *in vitro* detection gave a fair agreement (kappa 0.29), whereas comparison of PCR using gDNA and RT-PCR or *in vitro* detection resulted in a slight agreement (kappa 0.05 and 0.08, respectively) only. At 12 dpi, parasite gDNA was found in 10 out of 36 organs. In 7 of these organs viability of parasites was confirmed with NcGRA2-RT-PCR and growth of parasites in cell culture. Comparison of NcGRA2-RT-PCR and *in vitro* detection gave a substantial agreement (kappa 0.8), whereas comparison of PCR using gDNA and RT-PCR or *in vitro* detection resulted in a moderate agreement (kappa 0.59 and 0.77, respectively). As NcGRA2-RT-PCR is almost as sensitive as *in vitro* cultivation in detecting live parasites, it represents a fast, easy and safe method of viable parasite detection, and thus an attractive alternative to the *in vitro* cultivation approach.

**Key words**: *Neospora caninum*, NcGRA2-RT-PCR, *in vitro* inoculation

## Introduction

Currently, there is a generalized agreement on considering *Neospora caninum* as the protozoan pathogen which is most frequently associated with bovine abortion worldwide. The conventional diagnostic tools that have been made available so far, aimed at detecting the parasite and to discriminate *Neospora caninum* from infections with closely related parasites, such as *Toxoplasma gondii* or *Sarcocystis spp.*. Indirect techniques, based on serum antibody detection, prove parasite contact, but provide no information about the actual status of infection or disease, unless e.g. avidity is determined [1]. Direct detection techniques include histopathological investigations, complemented by molecular means such as the polymerase chain reaction (PCR) or by *in vitro* isolation of the parasite upon cell culture. Substantial efforts have been made to improve *N. caninum*-specific PCRs, which provide highly sensitive and specific parameters for the parasite detection by amplification of parasite specific sequences, such as the internal transcribed spacer 1 (ITS 1) [2] or a *Neospora*-specific genomic DNA (gDNA) sequence named Nc5 [3]. However, the presence of parasite gDNA in infected tissue does not necessarily provide information on the parasite viability. Thus, conventionally *in vivo* and *in vitro* tests are being used by inoculating appropriate samples into laboratory animals or cell culture [4]. Immunosuppressed mice, IFN-γ knock-out mice and gerbils (*Meriones unguiculatus*) are highly susceptible to *N. caninum* and were therefore used for corresponding tests [5-7]. The success of these methods strongly depends on the number of parasites and the state of the tissues. Especially in cell culture, opportunistic microbial contaminations are a big problem, as cultures have to be observed for a long time period.

Recently, we described a novel PCR that was established as a useful tool to distinguish between live and dead parasites in cell culture following a chemotherapeutic impairment of parasite viability [8]. NcGRA2-RT-PCR was specific for *N. caninum* and sensitive enough to detect 0.1 parasites equivalents per reaction [8]. In the present work, we compared the NcGRA2-RT-PCR for detection of live parasites *ex vivo* in organs from experimentally infected animals with the conventional approach to inoculate diagnostic material into appropriate cell culture subsequently maintained for 4 weeks.

## Materials and Methodology

### Tissue culture media, chemicals and drugs

If not otherwise stated, all tissue culture media were purchased from Gibco-BRL (Basel, Switzerland) and biochemical reagents were from Sigma (Buchs, Switzerland).

### Tissue culture and parasite purification

Cultures of Vero cells were maintained in RPMI 1640 medium (Gibco-BRL, Basel, Switzerland) supplemented with 5% fetal calf serum (FCS), 4 mM L-glutamine, 100 U/ml penicillin G, 100 µg/ml streptomycin and 0.25 µg/ml amphotericin B at 37 °C with 5% $CO_2$. Human foreskin fibroblasts (HFF) were maintained in Dulbecco`s modified Eagle`s medium (DMEM) containing the same additives and were identically treated. Cultures were trypsinized at least once a week. *N. caninum* (Nc-1 isolate) tachyzoites were maintained in Vero cell monolayer cultures, during which time FCS was replaced with immunoglobulin G-free horse serum (HS). Tachyzoites were harvested when they were still intracellular by trypsinization of infected Vero cells followed by repeated passage through a 25-gauge needle. Host cell debris were removed from the parasites by separation on Sephadex-G25 columns as previously described [9]. The tachyzoites were counted using a Neubauer chamber and parasite numbers were adjusted by adding RPMI medium as appropriate for experimental infection.

### Mice, infection, euthanasia and sample collection

12 wild-type C57BL/6 female mice were purchased from Charles River Laboratories (Sulzfeld, Germany) and randomly separated into two groups with 6 mice each. Food mix and water were provided *ad libitum*. All mice (10 weeks of age) were infected intraperitoneally (i.p.) with $1 \times 10^6$ live Nc-1 tachyzoites suspended in 200 µl RPMI medium at the same time point. Mice were daily checked for clinical signs. A group of 6 mice was euthanized by $CO_2$-inhalation 6 and 12 days post infection (dpi). From all animals, a brain hemisphere, the lungs, heart, liver, kidney and uterus were removed, disrupted with a scalpel blade and subsequently divided into three parts. Two parts were immediately frozen in liquid nitrogen and stored at -80 °C prior to gDNA and RNA isolation. A third part was suspended in 1 ml RPMI medium and transferred into

a falcon tube. The same volume of trypsin (0.05 % trypsin, 0.53 mM EDTA•4Na in hanks' balanced salt solution, Gibco-BRL) was added and the suspension was further disrupted with a syringe and needle starting from G18 to G23. The suspension was sedimented at 400 g to remove trypsin, and the remaining pellet was re-suspended in 4 ml DMEM medium containing 500 U/ml penicillin G, 500 µg/ml streptomycin, 1.25 µg/ml amphotericin B and 5% HS. Suspension was immediately used for inoculation of cell cultures.

**Inoculation of cell cultures**
HFF, as susceptible host cells, were grown to confluent monolayer in 24-well tissue culture plates, and subsequently inoculated with 1 ml of the diagnostic cell suspension per well. For each organ, 4 wells were inoculated with organ homogenates. The culture medium was changed after 24 h and then every second day. The cultures were daily checked for putatively growing parasites or contaminations. Cell cultures containing visible parasites and cultures grown for 4 weeks without visible parasites were lysed directly in the wells using 200 µl PBS containing Proteinase K (12 mAU/ml) and 200 µl AL buffer (DNeasy® blood and tissue kit; QIAGEN, Basel, Switzerland). Lysates were frozen at -80 °C prior to DNA purification.

**DNA extraction**
DNA purification from organs was performed using the DNeasy® blood and tissue kit (QIAGEN) according to the standard protocol suitable for animal tissues. Frozen organs were equilibrated to room temperature and lysed overnight at 56°C in ATL buffer containing Proteinase K (12 mAU/ml). DNA purification from cell lysates was performed using the DNeasy® blood and tissue kit (QIAGEN) according to the standard protocol suitable for animal blood or cells. Frozen lysates were equilibrated to room temperature before starting. gDNA was eluted in 100 µl AE buffer, boiled at 95 °C for 3 min and frozen at -80 °C prior to PCR.

**RNA extraction**
Total RNA isolation from brains was performed using the RNeasy® lipid tissue mini kit (QIAGEN) according to the standard protocol suitable for lipid animal tissues. Total RNA isolation from hearts and uteri was performed using the RNeasy® mini kit

(QIAGEN) according to the standard protocol suitable for heart, muscle and skin tissues. Total RNA isolation from lungs, livers and kidneys was performed using the RNeasy® mini kit (QIAGEN) according to the standard protocol suitable for animal tissues. All tissues were disrupted in the corresponding buffer with a small mortar. Except of the brain lysates, all lysates were loaded onto QIAshredder™ spin columns (QIAGEN) and centrifuged at maximum speed for 2 min after disruption. RNA purification included a DNA digestion step with RNase-free DNase (QIAGEN) for 1 h at room temperature. RNA was eluted in 60 µl RNase-free water, boiled at 95 °C for 3 min and immediately used for cDNA synthesis.

**Reverse Transcription**

RNA concentration was measured with the NanoDrop (Thermo Scientific, Delaware, US) system. cDNA synthesis was performed using the Omniscript® Reverse Transcription kit (QIAGEN) according to the standard protocol for first-strand cDNA synthesis. Briefly, 0.5 µg random Primer (Promega, Wallisellen, Switzerland) and 100 ng (uterus), 500 ng (lung, kidney, heart) or 1000 ng (brain, liver) of RNA were used in a final volume of 20 µl reaction mix and incubated for 1 h at 37 °C. cDNA was boiled at 95 °C for 3 min and frozen at -80 °C prior to PCR.

**Conventional PCR**

Detection of parasite-specific gDNA by Nc5-PCR was done as previously described [10] with *N. caninum*-specific primers Np21plus and Np6plus in a thermal cycler (Gene Amp PCR System model 9700; Applied Biosystems, Basel Switzerland). For the mix, 20 pmol of each primer and 1 µl DNA in a final volume of 25 µl were used.

Detection of parasite-specific cDNA by NcGRA2-RT-PCR was done as recently described [8] with *N. caninum*-specific primers NcGRA2-F1 and NcGRA2-R2. PCR was performed using 25 pmol of each primer and 1 µl cDNA in a final volume of 25 µl.

Both PCR-mixes were performed using the AmpliTaq® DNA polymerase kit (Applied Biosystems). To prevent carry-over contamination from previous reactions, the samples were incubated with uracyl DNA glycosylase (UDG; Roche Diagnostics, Basel, Switzerland) for 10 min at 20 °C. The UDG was inactivated by incubation at 95 °C for 2 min. Each run included a negative (water) and a positive (purified parasites) sample.

**Statistical analyses**

To measure the agreement between the methods, kappa statistic was used. Calculation and interpretation of kappa was performed as described by [11].

## Results

At 6 dpi, all of the 6 experimentally infected mice were devoid of any clinical signs. Following sacrifice, organs were removed from animals to extract gDNA and RNA, and to generate tissue cell suspension for inoculation onto host cell culture. Parasite gDNA was detected in 5 out of 6 brains, 6 out of 6 lungs, 6 out of 6 hearts, 5 out of 6 livers, 6 out of 6 kidneys and 6 out of 6 uteri from the group of experimentally infected animals. With the NcGRA2-RT-PCR, live parasites were detected in 2 out of 6 brains, 6 out of 6 lungs and 3 out of 6 hearts. NcGRA2-RT-PCR remained negative for all livers, kidneys and uteri of the same group of experimentally infected animals. Parasite proliferation was observed in HFF host cell culture inoculated with brains (2 out of 6), lungs (5 out of 6), hearts (1 out of 6), livers (2 out of 6), kidneys (1 out of 6) and uteri (4 out of 6) (Table 1). Parasites started to visibly (microscopy) grow in culture between 14 and 29 days after inoculation.

With *Neospora*-PCR using gDNA 34 out of 36 tested organs were *Neospora*-positive. In 7 out of 34 cases, we could prove with both NCGRA2-RT-PCR and *in vitro* cultivation, respectively, that parasites detected with conventional gDNA-PCR, actually were viable. In 15 organs, *Neospora*-gDNA was detected but viability of parasites could not be confirmed, neither by NcGRA2-RT-PCR nor by *in vitro* cultivation. Two organs were *N. caninum*-negative by all three methods. For 4 *Neospora*-gDNA positive organs, parasite viability was proven with NcGRA2RT-PCR only, whereas in another 8 organs parasite viability was shown in cell culture only. Comparison of viable parasite detection using RT-PCR or *in vitro* detection resulted in a fair agreement (kappa 0.29) with an observed agreement of 67% and an expected agreement of 53%. Slight agreements were observed when results of PCR using gDNA were compared with RT-PCR and *in vitro* detection (kappa 0.05 and 0.08, respectively).

By day 12 dpi, none of the infected mice showed any clinical signs due to neosporosis. All 6 mice were euthanized and organs were taken for gDNA and RNA extraction, and to obtain an organ cell suspension for subsequent diagnostic inoculation in host cell culture. Parasite gDNA was detected in 6 out of 6 brains, 1 out of 6 lungs and 3 out of 6 uteri, whereas no gDNA was found in hearts, livers and kidneys. With the NcGRA2-RT-PCR, live parasites were detected in 5 out of 6 brains, whereas all the other organs remained respectively negative. Upon *in vitro* cultivation, parasite proliferation was observed in host cell culture inoculated with brains (6 out of 6) and in 1 out of 6 uteri. No parasites were seen after 4 weeks in cultures inoculated with lungs, heart, livers and kidneys (Table 2). After inoculation in host cell culture, parasites started to grow between days 8 and 17.

In 5 *Neospora*-gDNA positive brains, parasite viability was observed by both, NCGRA2-RT-PCR and *in vitro* cultivation. For 2 *Neospora*-gDNA positive organs, we demonstrated parasite viability upon cell culture approach only. In 3 organs, although *Neospora*-gDNA was detected, a respective viability of parasites could not be confirmed, neither by NcGRA2-RT-PCR nor by *in vitro* cultivation. Furthermore, 26 out of 36 organs were negative for all three diagnostic methods.

Comparing RT-PCR and *in vitro* detection results, we observed an agreement of 94%. The agreement by chance was 72%. Kappa calculation gave a substantial agreement (kappa 0.8). PCR using gDNA compared with RT-PCR and *in vitro* detection resulted in a moderate agreement (kappa 0.59 and 0.77, respectively).

## Discussion and Conclusion

The availability of routine diagnostic tools to detect *N. caninum*-infections in animals prompted a more detailed approach, aimed at discriminating between alive and died-out parasites. Conventional tools such as serology, histopathology and PCR yield an etiological diagnosis, but no direct information on actual viability of parasites at the time point of collection of diagnostic samples. The only alternative so far consisted in diagnostic *in vivo* or *in vitro* cultivation of sample suspensions by using susceptible mice or cell culture. Such techniques may be valuable for research purposes, but for routine or mass investigations, they are tedious, time-consuming and expensive. Nevertheless, distinction between live and dead organisms is an important tool, for example, in testing chemotherapeutical efficacy or in assessing infectiosity of carrier animals or organs. Recently, a RT-PCR based on the *NcGRA2* gene was established in view to distinguish between parasiticidal and parasitostatic efficacy of given compounds in cell-culture-based assays [8].

In the present work, we used the same NcGRA2-RT-PCR to detect live parasites in organs obtained from experimentally *Neospora*-infected mice. To validate the results, we carried out parallel experiments by inoculating identical diagnostic materials into appropriate cell culture. In previous works, it was shown that at an early stage of infection, *N. caninum* can be detected in almost all organs of infected animals [12]. In the present study, mice examined at 6 dpi yielded similar findings, in that we revealed the presence of parasite-gDNA in almost all organs. Nevertheless, DNA does not automatically imply viable parasites, whereas RNA synthesis takes place only in live organisms. In the present study, only 19 out of 34 DNA-positive organs actually contained viable parasites as detected with NcGRA2-RT-PCR or *in vitro* cultivation or both, resulting in slight agreement only between DNA and viable parasite detection. During the course of infection, parasites may die due to host immune reactions or by other reasons, and DNA may still be present in affected organs, conversely to RNA that is much less stable. From 19 samples with live parasites, viable parasites were detected in 7 organs with both methods, NcGRA2-RT-PCR and *in vitro* cultivation. Here, lungs were the organs with the highest agreement. For other organs, either RT-PCR or *in vitro* cultivation gave a positive result, due to the fact that only few parasites were available in the corresponding organ and an unequal distribution during the experimental procedure. Nevertheless, results of RT-PCR and *in vitro* cultivation showed a fair agreement.

After the acute phase of infection, reflected by the presence of parasites in multiple organs, tachyzoites withdraw from most organs to switch into the brain, putatively related to the fact that this organ is less involved in systemic immune reactivity. In our experiment, at day 12 dpi, we preferentially found parasite-gDNA in the brain. Except of one brain, we could confirm with both viability tests that the gDNA belonged to live parasites. Substantial agreement was observed between RT-PCR and *in vitro* cultivation approach. Both viability tests never yielded a positive result when the PCR using gDNA was negative.

In comparison, NcGRA2-RT-PCR is as sensitive as *in vitro* detection of viable parasites, but RT-PCR is much faster and easier to handle than the *in vitro* cultivation. Especially for mass investigations, including a high number of tissue samples, RNA isolation and RT-PCR presents a fast method to detect remaining live parasites. Furthermore, there is less risk of sample contamination, especially if the PCR is done with material directly and freshly isolated from mouse tissue, this compared to culturing the materials for 4 weeks. The NcGRA2-RT-PCR appeared as a useful alternative tool to determine viability status of *N. caninum* in organs of infected animals. Distinction between live and dead parasites is important in treatment and vaccination studies, and RT-PCR provided a fast, easy and safe option for this purpose. The use of immunocompromised animals to detect viable parasites is the most sensitive technique so far. However, as detection of viable parasites in tissue from infected animals by NcGRA2-RT-PCR was tested for the first time, we used *in vitro* cultivation – in reference to [8] - to obtain information about sensitivity and handling procedure of the new technique. In a further future step, NcGRA2-RT-PCR will be compared with inoculation of diagnostic materials (obtained from naturally infected bovines) into immunocompromised mice.

## Acknowledgements

The study was supported by Bayer HealthCare AG (Leverkusen), the Swiss Federal Office of Science and Education (BBW C01.0122 in the frame of COST 854) and the Swiss National Foundation (SNF 3100A0-112532 / 1).

# References

[1] Aguado-Martinez A, Alvarez-Garcia G, Arnaiz-Seco I, Innes E, Ortega-Mora LM. Use of avidity enzyme-linked immunosorbent assay and avidity Western blot to discriminate between acute and chronic *Neospora caninum* infection in cattle. J Vet Diagn Invest 2005; 17(5): 442-50.

[2] Payne S, Ellis J. Detection of *Neospora caninum* DNA by the polymerase chain reaction. Int J Parasitol 1996; 26(4): 347-51.

[3] Kaufmann H, Yamage M, Roditi I, Dobbelaere D, Dubey JP, Holmdahl OJ, Trees A, Gottstein B. Discrimination of *Neospora caninum* from *Toxoplasma gondii* and other apicomplexan parasites by hybridization and PCR. Mol Cell Probes 1996; 10(4): 289-97.

[4] Dubey JP, Schares G, Ortega-Mora LM. Epidemiology and control of neosporosis and *Neospora caninum*. Clin Microbiol Rev 2007; 20(2): 323-67.

[5] Dubey JP, Lindsay DS. Gerbils (*Meriones unguiculatus*) are highly susceptible to oral infection with *Neospora caninum* oocysts. Parasitol Res 2000; 86(2): 165-8.

[6] Ramamoorthy S, Sriranganathan N, Lindsay DS. Gerbil model of acute neosporosis. Vet Parasitol 2005; 127(2): 111-4.

[7] Dubey JP, Dorough KR, Jenkins MC, Liddell S, Speer CA, Kwok OC, Shen SK. Canine neosporosis: clinical signs, diagnosis, treatment and isolation of *Neospora caninum* in mice and cell culture. Int J Parasitol 1998; 28(8): 1293-304.

[8] Strohbusch M, Müller N, Hemphill A, Greif G, Gottstein B. NcGRA2 as a molecular target to assess the parasiticidal activity of toltrazuril against *Neospora caninum*. Parasitology 2008; 135(9): 1065-73.

[9] Hemphill A, Gottstein B, Kaufmann H. Adhesion and invasion of bovine endothelial cells by *Neospora caninum*. Parasitology 1996; 112 (Pt 2): 183-97.

[10] Müller N, Zimmermann V, Hentrich B, Gottstein B. Diagnosis of *Neospora caninum* and *Toxoplasma gondii* infection by PCR and DNA hybridization immunoassay. J Clin Microbiol 1996; 34(11): 2850-2.

[11] Viera AJ, Garrett JM. Understanding interobserver agreement: The kappa statistic. Fam Med 2005; 37(5): 360-3.

[12] Collantes-Fernàndez E, Lopez-Perez I, Alvarez-Garcia G, Ortega-Mora LM. Temporal distribution and parasite load kinetics in blood and tissues during *Neospora caninum* infection in mice. Infect Immun 2006; 74(4): 2491-4.

**Legends to Tables**

**Table 1**

*Neospora caninum* detection 6 days post infection.

*Neospora caninum* was detected by three different methods (PCR based on gDNA or cDNA and *in vitro* cultivation) in a group of six mice experimentally infected with *N. caninum* tachyzoites. Animals were investigated 6 days post infection.

¤ all detection methods negative

+ all detection methods positive

+ positive result

- negative result


**Table 2**

*Neospora caninum* detection 12 days post infection.

*Neospora caninum* was detected by three different methods (PCR based on gDNA or cDNA and *in vitro* cultivation) in a group of six mice experimentally infected with *N. caninum* tachyzoites. Animals were investigated 12 days post infection.

¤ all detection methods negative

+ all detection methods positive

+ positive result

- negative result

Tab. 1

|  | Mouse 1 | | | Mouse 2 | | | Mouse 3 | | | Mouse 4 | | | Mouse 5 | | | Mouse 6 | | |
|---|---|---|---|---|---|---|---|---|---|---|---|---|---|---|---|---|---|---|
|  | gDNA | cDNA | in vitro | gDNA | cDNA | in vitro | gDNA | cDNA | in vitro | gDNA | cDNA | in vitro | gDNA | cDNA | in vitro | gDNA | cDNA | in vitro |
| Brain | + | + | + | + | - | - | □ | □ | □ | + | - | - | + | - | + | + | + | - |
| Lung | + | + | + | + | + | + | + | + | + | + | + | + | + | + | + | + | + | - |
| Heart | + | + | + | + | - | - | + | + | - | + | + | - | + | - | - | + | - | - |
| Liver | + | - | - | + | - | + | + | - | - | + | - | + | + | - | - | □ | □ | □ |
| Kidney | + | - | - | + | - | - | + | - | - | + | - | + | + | - | - | + | - | - |
| Uterus | ! | - | - | ! | - | ! | ! | - | - | ! | - | ! | ! | - | ! | ! | - | ! |

Tab. 2

|  | Mouse 7 | | | Mouse 8 | | | Mouse 9 | | | Mouse 10 | | | Mouse 11 | | | Mouse 12 | | |
|---|---|---|---|---|---|---|---|---|---|---|---|---|---|---|---|---|---|---|
|  | gDNA | cDNA | in vitro | gDNA | cDNA | in vitro | gDNA | cDNA | in vitro | gDNA | cDNA | in vitro | gDNA | cDNA | in vitro | gDNA | cDNA | in vitro |
| Brain | + | - | + | + | + | + | + | + | + | + | + | + | + | + | + | + | + | + |
| Lung | □ | □ | □ | + |  |  | □ | □ | □ | □ | □ | □ | □ | □ | □ | □ | □ | □ |
| Heart | □ | □ | □ | □ | □ | □ | □ | □ | □ | □ | □ | □ | □ | □ | □ | □ | □ | □ |
| Liver | □ | □ | □ | □ | □ | □ | □ | □ | □ | □ | □ | □ | □ | □ | □ | □ | □ | □ |
| Kidney | □ | □ | □ | □ | □ | □ | □ | □ | □ | □ | □ | □ | □ | □ | □ | □ | □ | □ |
| Uterus | □ | □ | □ | + | - | - | + | - | - | + | - | + | □ | □ | □ | □ | □ | □ |

# Manuscripts

**Toltrazuril treatment of congenitally acquired *Neospora caninum*-infection in newborn mice**

Maria Strohbusch[1], Norbert Müller[1], Andrew Hemphill[1], Gisela Greif[2], Bruno Gottstein[1]*

[1]Institute of Parasitology, University of Berne, Laenggass-Strasse 122, CH-3012 Bern, Switzerland
[2]Bayer HealthCare AG, Leverkusen, Germany

*address for correspondence:

Institute of Parasitology
Vetsuisse Faculty
University of Bern
Laenggassstrasse 122
CH-3001 Bern, Switzerland
+41 31 631 24 18
bruno.gottstein@ipa.unibe.ch

## Abstract

In the present study, mice were infected with *N. caninum* tachyzoites during pregnancy, yielding a transplacental infection of developing foetuses. Subsequently, congenitally infected newborn mice were treated either once or three-times with toltrazuril or a corresponding placebo. These treatments had no negative effect on newborns as non-infected treated pups developed normal without differences in mortality and morbidity. Already one application of toltrazuril was able to delay the outbreak of neosporosis in newborn mice significantly ($p < 0.01$). Those toltrazuril-treated pups that diseased did this, independent of the dosage schedule, at significant ($p < 0.01$) later time points than corresponding placebo-treated animals. We found significantly higher survival rates in one-time and three-time-toltrazuril-treated pups (34.5%; 53.6%) compared to one-time- and three-time-placebo-treated pups (13.6%; 30.4%), respectively. There was no significant difference ($p = 0.2$) in the survival rates between one- and three-time-toltrazuril treatment. However, the number of diseased and *Neospora*-positive pups (46.4% and 46.7%, respectively), was markedly reduced after three-time-toltrazuril-treatment compared to all other groups. Three-time-treatment also resulted in the highest antibody (IgG, IgG2a) response.

All in all, we could show that treatment with three applications of toltrazuril can influence the course of infection in congenitally *N. caninum*-infected newborn mice.

**Key words**: *Neospora caninum*, neosporosis, toltrazuril, pregnancy

## Introduction

The main problems associated with *N. caninum* and the corresponding disease, neosporosis, are (i) abortion in cattle (Dubey 2003), causing serious veterinary health issues and economic losses within livestock production (Hemphill and Gottstein 2000; Dubey, Schares et al. 2007), and (ii) neuromuscular disease in dogs (Dubey, 2003).

The need for the development of effective pro- or metaphylactic measures against bovine neosporosis has been widely addressed and discussed (Liddell, Jenkins et al. 1999; Gottstein, Eperon et al. 2001; Innes, Andrianarivo et al. 2002; Kritzner, Sager et al. 2002; Häsler, Regula et al. 2006; Häsler, Stärk et al. 2006). Although there are successful experimental vaccination approaches to prevent cerebral neosporosis (Cannas, Naguleswaran et al. 2003; Cannas, Naguleswaran et al. 2003) or vertical transmission (Nishikawa, Xuan et al. 2001) in mice, there are currently no vaccines available to protect cattle from abortion (Andrianarivo, Rowe et al. 2000; Innes and Vermeulen 2006).

Chemotherapy is being discussed as an interesting alternative to the vaccination strategy. So far, a wide range of compounds have been tested in cell culture-based assays and some pharmacologically active compounds, including lasalocid, monensin, piritrexim, pyrimethamine and trimethoprim, were found to exhibit parasiticidal activity against *N. caninum* (Lindsay and Dubey 1989; Lindsay, Rippey et al. 1994). More recently, it was reported that nitazoxanide (NTZ) and a series of NTZ-derivatives efficiently inhibited *N. caninum* proliferation (Esposito, Stettler et al. 2005; Esposito, Moores et al. 2006; Esposito, Müller et al. 2007). *In vivo* studies showed that oral drug treatment of *Neospora*-infected mice with sulfadiazine and amprolium was rather ineffective (Lindsay and Dubey 1990).

Toltrazuril, a symmetric triazinon derivative, was shown to exhibit anti-coccidial activity against cyst-forming and non-cyst-forming coccidian parasites (Haberkorn 1996). The effect(s) of toltrazuril on the fine structure and multiplication of *N. caninum* were studied in cell culture demonstrating lethal damage in *N. caninum* tachyzoites (Darius, Mehlhorn et al. 2004). The effect of toltrazuril on parasite survival after long-term treatments in cell culture, assessed by quantitative-RT PCR, revealed a parasiticidal activity starting after a continuous 14-day treatment (Strohbusch, Müller et al. 2008). In the murine model of experimental *N. caninum* infection, toltrazuril treatment prevented severe clinical signs and formation of cerebral lesions (Gottstein, Eperon et al. 2001; Darius, Mehlhorn et al. 2004). However, an efficient metaphylaxis required at least a T-cell-mediated immunological support in mice (Ammann, Waldvogel et al. 2004). It was also reported that toltrazuil-treatment of an acute *N. caninum* infection – induced during pregnancy in mice – resulted in a significant reduction of foetal losses (Gottstein, Razmi et al. 2005). Furthermore, initially explorative approaches indicated a basic effectiveness of toltrazuril and its major metabolite, ponazuril, against experimental *N. caninum* infection in calves (Kritzner, Sager et al. 2002; Härdi, Hässig et al. 2006).

In this study we used the mouse model to determine whether treatment of neonates with toltrazuril has any effect, positive or negative on outcome of disease and infection.

## Material and Methods

### Tissue culture media, biochemicals and drugs
If not otherwise stated, all tissue culture media were purchased from Gibco-BRL (Basel, Switzerland) and biochemical reagents were from Sigma (St. Louis, MO, US). Toltrazuril and the corresponding placebo formulated for oral application were provided by Bayer HealthCare AG (Germany), stock solutions were diluted with water and used immediately.

### Tissue culture and parasite purification
Cultures of Vero cells were maintained in RPMI 1640 medium (Gibco-BRL, Basel, Switzerland) supplemented with 5% fetal calf serum (FCS), 4 mM L-glutamine, 100 U/ml penicillin G, 100 µg/ml streptomycin and 0.25 µg/ml amphotericin B at 37°C with 5% $CO_2$. Cultures were trypsinized at least once a week. *N. caninum* (Nc-1 isolate) tachyzoites were maintained in Vero cell monolayer cultures, during which time FCS was replaced with immunoglobulin G-free horse serum. Tachyzoites were harvested when they were still intracellular by trypsinization of infected Vero cells followed by repeated passage through a 25-gauge needle. Host cell debris were removed from parasites by separation on Sephadex-G25 columns as previously described (Hemphill, Gottstein et al. 1996). The tachyzoites were counted using a Neubauer chamber and parasite numbers were adjusted by adding RPMI medium as appropriate for experimental infection.

### Mice, infection, treatment and euthanasia
21 pregnant wild-type C57BL/6 mice were purchased from Charles River Laboratories (Sulzfeld, Germany) at gestation day (GD) 13 and were infected with *N. caninum* or medium immediately upon arrival. Mice were maintained under conventional day/night-cycle housing conditions as required by the animal welfare legislation of the Swiss Veterinary Office. Special food mix for breeding mice and water were provided *ad libitum*. For infection, 18 mice were randomly selected and infected intraperitoneally (i.p.) with $6 \times 10^5$ live NC-1 tachyzoites suspended in 200 µl RPMI medium. Control mice (n = 3) received 200 µl medium without parasites. Mice were individually housed and checked daily for clinical signs, abortion or preterm birth. Day of delivery was designated as day 0. Newborn mice were counted and

daily checked for survival and health status. Infected dams and corresponding litters were randomly selected and divided into four treatment groups (groups C – F). Neonates from infected dams were treated either once (group C) or three-times (group D) with toltrazuril, or once (group E) or three-times (group F) with placebo, respectively. Newborns from uninfected control mice were treated three-times with toltrazuril (group A) or placebo (group B). The first dose was administered on two following days. Toltrazuril at a concentration of 31.25 mg/kg body weight (bw), or the same dilution of placebo, was applied at day 3 and 4 of age, respectively. The treatment was done orally using a pipette, taking advantage of the sucking effect of newborns. Treatments were repeated identically at days 14 and 29 with 62.5 mg/kg bw. Cages were daily checked and dead pups, if found, were removed as soon as possible. Pups and dams with clinical signs were euthanized immediately by $CO_2$-inhalation. All other dams were separated from pups and euthanized at day 28 (33dpi), remaining pups were euthanized between day 64 and 100 of age. From all animals, pieces of brain, lung, heart, and liver were collected and stored at -20°C prior to DNA extraction. If possible, blood was taken for ELISA.

**Vertical transmission**

The vertical transmission rate from infected dams to foetuses was calculated retrospectively. All pups that died before the treatment started and pups from infected and placebo-treated groups (E, F) were tested for *Neospora*-infection by conventional PCR (see below). The number of PCR-positive pups was divided by the overall number of pups from these groups.

**DNA extraction**

DNA purification was performed using the DNeasy blood and tissue kit (QIAGEN, Basel, Switzerland) according to the standard protocol suitable for animal tissues. Frozen organs were equilibrate to room temperature and then lysed overnight at 56°C in ATL buffer containing Proteinase K (12 mIAU/ml). DNA was eluted in 100 µl AE buffer, boiled at 95°C for 3 min and frozen at -80°C prior to PCR.

**Conventional PCR**

Detection of parasite-specific DNA by PCR was done as previously described (Müller, Zimmermann et al. 1996) with *N. caninum*-specific primers Np21plus and

Np6plus in a thermal cycler (Gene Amp PCR System model 9700; Applied Biosystems, Basel Switzerland). For the mix, 20 pmol of each primer and 1 µl DNA in a final volume of 25 µl were used. The PCR was performed using the AmpliTaq® DNA polymerase kit (Applied Biosystems). To prevent carry-over contamination from previous reactions, the samples were incubated with uracyl DNA glycosylase (UDG; Roche Diagnostics, Basel, Switzerland) for 10 min at 20°C. The UDG was inactivated by incubation at 95°C for 2 min. Each run included a negative (water) and a positive (purified parasites) probe as controls.

**Serology**

Mouse sera were analyzed for the presence of antibodies against Nc-1 antigen by enzyme-linked immunosorbent assay (ELISA) using the same somatic antigen as previously described (Eperon, Brönnimann et al. 1999). Alkaline-phosphate conjugated goat anti-mouse IgG (Promega, Duebendorf, Switzerland), anti-IgG1 or anti-IgG2a (both from Southern Biotechnology Associates, Birmingham, US) were used as second antibody (conjugate). Absorbance was measured at 405 nm ($A_{405}$, reference filter 630 nm) using a Dynatech MR 7000 ELISA reader and the corresponding Dynatech Biocalc software (Dynatech, Embrach, Switzerland). The threshold value arbitrarily discriminating between "positive" and "negative" (cut-off) was defined by adding three standard deviations to the mean $A_{405}$ value of the sera from non-infected and non-treated control mice.

**Statistical analyses**

Comparison of the IgG1 and IgG2a response in infected dams and number of eaten pups in the non-infected and infected groups were done using the student`s t-test. Specific antibody responses (IgG, IgG1, IgG2a) of the pups and the outbreak of the disease were analysed using one-way analysis of variance (ANOVA). A nonparametric Kruskal-Wallis test was used wherever the distributional assumptions required for an ANOVA were felt to be unrealistic. When statistical differences were found, a nonparametric multiple comparison test was used to examine all possible pair wise comparisons. Survival curves were calculated using the Kaplan-Meier-survival statistic and differences between groups were determined using the log-rank-survival tests. Pups that died or became ill during the experiment were designed as failed, healthy pups were designed as sensored. Differences between the numbers of diseased or PCR positive pups were analyzed by the chi-square test. A value of $p < 0.05$ was considered statistically significant. All statistical analyses were carried out using NCSS software version 2001 (NCSS, Kaysville, Utah).

## Results

### Infection of the dams and outcome of pregnancy

After infection at GD 13, none of control (n=3) and infected (n=18) dams showed abortion. All dams gave birth between GD 17 and 19. There was no difference (p = 0.2) in the number of pups per litter between uninfected and infected animals (Tab. 1). Three out of 18 infected dams became sick at day 19, 21 and 26 post infection, respectively. These three mice and also dams from which all pups died before the end of the lactation period (n = 4; 6, 11, 13, 21dpi), were sacrificed. Remaining infected (n = 11) and control (n = 3) dams were sacrificed at the end of the weaning period (33dpi corresponding to 28 days after delivery). All dams yielded positive (conventional) PCR-findings for *Neospora*-DNA in the brain (data not shown). Furthermore, all 18 infected dams were seropositive at necropsy as shown by *N. caninum*-ELISA. Investigation for immunoglobulin isotypes by ELISA revealed a significantly higher level of IgG2a than of IgG1 (p = 0.006) in infected dams (Fig. 1), indicating a rather Th1-oriented immune response after infection at GD 13. Uninfected control dams were all PCR-negative and *N. caninum*-ELISA seronegative.

### Treatment and subsequent survival rate of the newborn mice

All treated pups were daily checked for their health status. Pups eaten by the dam were excluded from further investigations. There was no significant difference in the number of eaten pups from uninfected or infected dams (p = 0.15). At day 3 of age, pups from uninfected dams were separated into two groups and treated either three-times with toltrazuril (A, n = 13) or three-times with placebo (B, n = 6). Chemotherapy itself with three temporally sequential applications of toltrazuril had no negative effect on health status and survival rates of the newborn pups, as uninfected control group (A) developed normally and showed no spontaneous morbidity and mortality after the last treatment until the end of the experiment.

Also at day three of age, pups from infected dams were separated in four different groups and treated as described in Tab. 2. When comparing survival rates of different infected treatment groups (C-F), significantly higher survival rates were found for toltrazuril-treated groups (Fig. 2). The survival rate of three-time-toltrazuril-treated pups (D) was significantly higher than the survival rate for three-time-placebo-treated ones (F) (53.6% vs 30.4%; p = 0.0072). A significant difference in the survival rates was also found between one-time-toltrazuril (C) and one-time-placebo (E) treated pups (34.5% vs 13.6%; p < 0.01). Nevertheless, there was no significant difference between the toltrazuril treatment groups C and D (p = 0.2), but three-time-toltrazuril treatment resulted in a 1.6 time higher survival rate compared to one-time-toltrazuril treatment (Tab. 2 + Fig 2).

## Outcome of disease

The outcome of disease in very young diseased animals was characterized by spontaneous death. Older pups showed typical signs of murine neosporosis (apathy, bent back, rough hair coat) and were euthanized at the time the symptoms appeared. Infected and placebo-treated pups (group E, n = 19; group F, n = 16) died or became sick within the first 27 days after birth. Most of infected and toltrazuril-treated pups (C, n = 19; D, n = 13), on the other hand, started to die or to show clinical signs from day 27 onwards (Fig. 3). This delay in the outbreak of neosporosis was significant (p < 0.01) between toltrazuril- and placebo-treated groups but not between the two toltrazuril-treated groups with different application schemes.

## Detection of *N. caninum* in congenitally infected and treated mice

Detection of parasite DNA was performed by PCR using DNA extracted from different organs of pups. The transmission, calculated retrospectively, revealed a vertical infection rate of 73.6%. The rate of PCR-positive pups in placebo-treated groups (E, F) ranged between 86.36% and 65.2%, whereas the rate of positive pups in toltrazuril-treated groups (C, D) was between 65.5% and 46.6% (Tab. 3). The difference in the number of PCR-positive pups was significant between the placebo- and toltrazuril-treated groups (p = 0.03). There was no significant difference, however, between one-time- and three-time-toltrazuril-treated pups (p = 0.14). We observed that those pups that became ill or died, independently of the treatment scheme, all had PCR-positive brains.

## Serological examination of congenitally infected mice

For serological studies, healthy pups sacrificed at the end of the experiment and pups prematurely sacrificed because of illness could be investigated. Pups that became ill during the experiment showed significantly (p < 0.01) higher IgG levels than pups that survived until the end of the experiment, independently of the treatment schedule (Fig. 4a). As healthy pups exhibited negative or only very low antibody levels, they were not included anymore for further data analyses. Comparison of the IgG levels of only diseased pups, taking into account the different treatment groups, revealed a significantly higher antibody response for three-time-toltrazuril-treated pups (D vs C, $p = 0.02$; D vs E, $p = 0.03$) (Fig. 4b). We also determined the main IgG-isotypes of diseased pups involved in the anti-*N. caninum* response. With regard to IgG1, there was no significant difference in antibody levels between the different treatment groups ($p = 0.08$) (Fig. 4c). With regard to IgG2a, there was a significantly higher respective antibody level in group D when compared to group C ($p = 0.007$) and group E ($p = 0.03$) (Fig. 4d). Finally, there were no significant differences between IgG1 and IgG2a levels when comparing results of different treatment groups. Consequently, this indicated that pups appeared to have mounted a mixed Th1/Th2 immune response following an *in utero* infection, independently of the treatment schedule subsequent to delivery.

## Discussion

To date, the main mode of control of neosporosis is based upon culling persistently infected, sero-positive reproducing animals, as there is no effective treatment for cattle available (Andrianarivo, Rowe et al. 2000; Innes and Vermeulen 2006). Toltrazuril is one of those few compounds that have demonstrated anti-parasitic activity against *N. caninum* infections not only in cell culture-based assays, but also in experimentally infected mice and even cattle (Darius, Mehlhorn et al. 2004a,b; Gottstein, Eperon et al. 2001; Gottstein, Razmi et al. 2005; Kritzner, Sager et al. 2002; Härdi, Hässig et al. 2006).

This study is a further step in assessing efficacy of toltrazuril, by addressing the effect of toltrazuril in congenitally *N. caninum* infected newborn mice. These experiments were intended to provide baseline data in a small animal model, prior to carrying out similar future experiments in the bovine system. Congenitally infected newborn mice were treated with toltrazuril right after birth, either once, or by three treatments. Control analyses showed that three consecutive applications of toltrazuril had no negative effect on development and health status of newborns. In order to provide an appropriate and constant high toltrazuril concentration in mice for at least 14 days, repeated applications of toltrazuril seemed to be necessary. Preliminary explorative experiments in cattle revealed a half-life time of the active substance in the serum of about 10 days (Kritzner, Sager et al. 2002). Furthermore, cell-culture-assays showed that toltrazuril required 14 days of *in vitro* treatment to yield parasiticidal activity; short-time exposures did not kill all parasites (Strohbusch, Müller et al. 2008). Both, one and three toltrazuril applications, significantly delayed the outbreak of neosporosis in newborn mice, as pups treated once or three-times with toltrazuril diseased at a significantly later age compared to placebo-treated pups. A marked delay of disease after toltrazuril treatment had already been observed in *N. caninum*-infected athymic nu⁻/nu⁻ mice, and these experiments had indicated that toltrazuril has a parasitostatic rather than a parasiticidal effect, requiring T-cell-mediated support to control neosporosis (Ammann, Waldvogel et al. 2004). In the present study, the overall survival rate of three-time-toltrazuril-treated pups was 1.6 times higher than the rate of one-time-treated pups. Consequently, one application of toltrazuril appeared not as effective as repeated treatment. Similar findings were observed when comparing the number of diseased pups or the number of *N.*

*caninum* PCR-positive pups. Both parameters were markedly reduced in three-time-toltrazuril-treated group compared to one-time-toltrazuril-treated and the placebo-treated pups.

It was shown earlier that newborn mice were as effective as adults in developing primary antigen-specific T-cell population within the first week of life (Adkins and Du 1998) and are thus fully immune competent at this age (Morein, Abusugra et al. 2002), although pathogen-specific immunity needs to be primarily developed upon first contact with respective organisms. Applied to our experiments, this allows the conclusion that congenitally infected pups appeared to have mounted a T-cell immune response supporting toltrazuril treatment effectively. Antibodies also play an important role in the control of *N. caninum*-infection, as B-cell deficient (µMT) mice were highly susceptible to infection (Eperon, Brönnimann et al. 1999). Our data revealed that three-time-toltrazuril treatment yielded the highest antibody responses in treated pups. This is in line with the findings of Härdi et al. (2006), who observed the development of a strong humoral immune response after toltrazuril chemotherapy of congenitally (naturally) infected calves (Härdi, Hässig et al. 2006). Similar results have also been documented in studies with *Eimeria*-infected chicken, where an increase of parasite-specific antibody response after toltrazuril-treatment was observed (Greif 2000).

The results presented in this study indicated that treatment with three applications of toltrazuril had the best positive effect to control the course of infection in congenitally *N. caninum*-infected newborn mice. The present application protocol could be a useful tool to address the question of efficacy in the experimental bovine model. Based on presumable level of efficacy, the final aim will be to develop an appropriate treatment schedule that allows controlling the problem at a national level with a positive cost-benefit ratio as claimed by Häsler et al. (2007).

Treatment of congenitally infected neonates would result in parasite-free breeding lines and reduce the prevalence of infection and/or disease within the herd. Because of the lower body weight of newborns, a lower amount of drug is needed and this would lower costs. Furthermore, withdrawal time with respect to meat and milk production would not be a problem.

## Acknowledgements

The study was supported by and Bayer HealthCare AG (Leverkusen), the Swiss Federal Office of Science and Education (BBW C01.0122 in the frame of COST 854) and the Swiss National Foundation (SNF 3100A0-112532 / 1).

## References

Adkins, B. and R. Q. Du (1998). "Newborn mice develop balanced Th1/Th2 primary effector responses in vivo but are biased to Th2 secondary responses." J Immunol 160(9): 4217-24.

Ammann, P., A. Waldvogel, et al. (2004). "The role of B- and T-cell immunity in toltrazuril-treated C57BL/6 WT, microMT and nude mice experimentally infected with *Neospora caninum*." Parasitol Res 93(3): 178-87.

Andrianarivo, A. G., J. D. Rowe, et al. (2000). "A POLYGEN-adjuvanted killed *Neospora caninum* tachyzoite preparation failed to prevent foetal infection in pregnant cattle following i.v./i.m. experimental tachyzoite challenge." Int J Parasitol 30(9): 985-90.

Cannas, A., A. Naguleswaran, et al. (2003). "Vaccination of mice against experimental *Neospora caninum* infection using NcSAG1- and NcSRS2-based recombinant antigens and DNA vaccines." Parasitology 126(Pt 4): 303-12.

Cannas, A., A. Naguleswaran, et al. (2003). "Reduced cerebral infection of *Neospora caninum*-infected mice after vaccination with recombinant microneme protein NcMIC3 and ribi adjuvant." J Parasitol 89(1): 44-50.

Darius, A. K., H. Mehlhorn, et al. (2004). "Effects of toltrazuril and ponazuril on *Hammondia heydorni* (syn. *Neospora caninum*) infections in mice." Parasitol Res 92(6): 520-2.

Darius, A. K., H. Mehlhorn, et al. (2004). "Effects of toltrazuril and ponazuril on the fine structure and multiplication of tachyzoites of the NC-1 strain *of Neospora caninum* (a synonym of *Hammondia heydorni*) in cell cultures." Parasitol Res 92(6): 453-8.

Dubey, J. P. (2003). "Review of *Neospora caninum* and neosporosis in animals." Kor J Parasitol 41(1): 1-16.

Dubey, J. P., G. Schares, et al. (2007). "Epidemiology and control of neosporosis and *Neospora caninum*." Clin Microbiol Rev 20(2): 323-367.

Eperon, S., K. Brönnimann, et al. (1999). "Susceptibility of B-cell deficient C57BL/6 (microMT) mice to *Neospora caninum* infection." Parasite Immunol 21(5): 225-36.

Esposito, M., S. L. Moores, et al. (2006). "Nitazoxanide and thiazolides, a novel class of broadspectrum anti-parasitic drugs." Res Adv Antimicrobial Agents Chemother 6: 1-11.

Esposito, M., N. Müller, et al. (2007). "Structure-activity relationships from in vitro efficacies of the thiazolide series against the intracellular apicomplexan protozoan Neospora caninum." Int J Parasitol 37(2): 183-90.

Esposito, M., R. Stettler, et al. (2005). "In vitro efficacies of nitazoxanide and other thiazolides against Neospora caninum tachyzoites reveal antiparasitic activity independent of the nitro group." Antimicrob Agents Chemother 49(9): 3715-23.

Gottstein, B., S. Eperon, et al. (2001). "Efficacy of toltrazuril and ponazuril against experimental Neospora caninum infection in mice." Parasitol Res 87(1): 43-8.

Gottstein, B., G. R. Razmi, et al. (2005). "Toltrazuril treatment to control diaplacental Neospora caninum transmission in experimentally infected pregnant mice." Parasitology 130(Pt 1): 41-8.

Greif, G. (2000). "Immunity to coccidiosis after treatment with toltrazuril." Parasitol Res 86: 787-790.

Haberkorn, A. (1996). "Chemotherapy of human and animal coccidioses: state and perspectives." Parasitol Res 82(3): 193-199.

Härdi, C., M. Hässig, et al. (2006). "Humoral immune reaction of newborn calves congenitally infected with Neospora caninum and experimentally treated with toltrazuril." Parasitol Res 99(5): 534-40.

Häsler, B., G. Regula, et al. (2006). "Financial analysis of various strategies for the control of Neospora caninum in dairy cattle in Switzerland." Prev. Vet. Med 77: 230-253.

Häsler, B., K. D. C. Stärk, et al. (2006). "Simultaing the impact of four control strategies on the population dynamics of Neospora caninum infection in Swiss dairy cattle." Prev. Vet. Med 77: 254-283.

Hemphill, A. and B. Gottstein (2000). "A European perspective on Neospora caninum." Int J Parasitol 30(8): 877-924.

Hemphill, A., B. Gottstein, et al. (1996). "Adhesion and invasion of bovine endothelial cells by Neospora caninum." Parasitology 112 (Pt 2): 183-97.

Innes, E. A., A. G. Andrianarivo, et al. (2002). "Immune responses to Neospora caninum and prospects for vaccination." Trends Parasitol 18(11): 497-504.

Innes, E. A. and A. N. Vermeulen (2006). "Vaccination as a control strategy against the coccidial parasites *Eimeria, Toxoplasma and Neospora*." Parasitology 133 Suppl: S145-68.

Kritzner, S., H. Sager, et al. (2002). "An explorative study to assess the efficacy of toltrazuril-sulfone (ponazuril) in calves experimentally infected with *Neospora caninum*." Ann Clin Microbiol Antimicrob 1: 4.

Liddell, S., M. C. Jenkins, et al. (1999). "Prevention of vertical transfer of *Neospora caninum* in BALB/c mice by vaccination." J Parasitol 85(6): 1072-5.

Lindsay, D. S. and J. P. Dubey (1989). "Evaluation of anti-coccidial drugs' inhibition of *Neospora caninum* development in cell cultures." J Parasitol 75(6): 990-2.

Lindsay, D. S. and J. P. Dubey (1990). "Effects of sulfadiazine and amprolium on *Neospora caninum* (Protozoa: Apicomplexa) infection in mice." J Parasitol 76: 177-179.

Lindsay, D. S., N. S. Rippey, et al. (1994). "Examination of the activities of 43 chemotherapeutic agents against *Neospora caninum* tachyzoites in cultured cells." Am J Vet Res 55(7): 976-81.

Moreln, B., I. Abusugra, et al. (2002). "Immunity in neoantes." Vet Immunol Immunopathol 87: 207-213.

Müller, N., V. Zimmermann, et al. (1996). "Diagnosis of *Neospora caninum* and *Toxoplasma gondii* infection by PCR and DNA hybridization immunoassay." J Clin Microbiol 34(11): 2850-2852.

Nishikawa, Y., X. Xuan, et al. (2001). "Prevention of vertical transmission of *Neospora caninum* in BALB/c mice by recombinant vaccinia virus carrying NcSRS2 gene." Vaccine 19(13-14): 1710-6.

Strohbusch, M., N. Müller, et al. (2008). "NcGRA2 as a molecular target to assess the parasiticidal activity of toltrazuril against *Neospora caninum*." Parasitology 135(9): 1065-73.

## Legends to Tables and Figures

### Table 1
Number of delivering dams and delivered newborns.
\# Total number of live newborns at day 0 (day of birth).
\* Number of pups that died before treatment, which started at day three of age. Pups were signed as untreated pups.
$ Number of pups that were eaten by mothers before or after treatment. These pups were logically excluded from the study because examinations were not possible.

### Table 2
Number of pups in different treatment groups at beginning and at the end of the treatment study.
\# Number of pups included in the study. Eaten pups are not mentioned.
\* Survival rate of pups, calculated with Kaplan-Meier-survival statistics.

### Table 3
Number of PCR-positive pups in different treatment groups. PCR was performed with organs from all of these pups.

### Figure 1
Anti-*N. caninum* IgG-isotype levels of infected dams as determined by ELISA. There was a significantly higher IgG2a level compared to IgG1 level in these dams. Significance hold true when $p < 0.05$ (*).

### Figure 2
Survival rates of pups. Survival rates were calculated with Kaplan-Meier-survival statistics. Untreated and eaten pups were excluded. Pups that died or became ill during the experiment were designed as failed, healthy pups were designed as sensored. Statistical differences were calculated with log-rank-survival tests. Significant differences (* $p < 0.05$) were found between the survival rates of one- and three-times-toltrazuril-treated pups compared with one- and three-times-placebo-treated pups, but not between one- and three-times-toltrazuril-treated pups.

**Figure 3**

Outbreak of disease depended on the age of pups. Outbreak of disease was defined when a pup died or became ill and was tested positive by *Neospora*-PCR. There was a significant difference in the age when pups became ill between toltrazuril and placebo treated pups. Significance hold true when $p < 0.05$ (*).

**Figure 4**

Antibody response of pups from infected dams. (A) Comparison of IgG levels between pups that became ill during the experiment and pups those were healthy at the end of the experiment. There was a significant difference between the two groups. (B) Comparison of IgG levels between diseased pups of different treatment groups. There was a significant difference between three-times-toltrazuril-treated pups and all other groups. (C) Comparison of the IgG1 level between diseased pups of different treatment groups. There was no difference between the two treatment groups. (D) Comparison of the IgG2a level between diseased pups of different treatment groups. There was a significant difference between three-times-toltrazuril treated pups and all other groups. Significance hold true when $p < 0.05$ (*).

Tab. 1

|  | con | inf |
|---|---|---|
| No. of delivering dams | 3/3 | 21/21 |
| Average pups/litter | 8.6 (7, 10) | 7.2 (3, 10) |
| Total no. of newborns # | 26 | 130 |
| Died before treatment * | 0 | 8 |
| Eaten during experiment $ | 7 | 20 |

Tab. 2

| treatment group | 1xPla | 3xPla | 1xTol | 3xTol |
|---|---|---|---|---|
| N° start # | 22 | 23 | 29 | 28 |
| Survival (end) * | 13.6% | 30.4% | 34.5% | 53.6% |

Tab. 3

|  | 1xPla | 3xPla | 1xTol | 3xTol |
|---|---|---|---|---|
| PCR+ | 86.36% | 65.2% | 65.5% | 46.7% |

Fig. 1

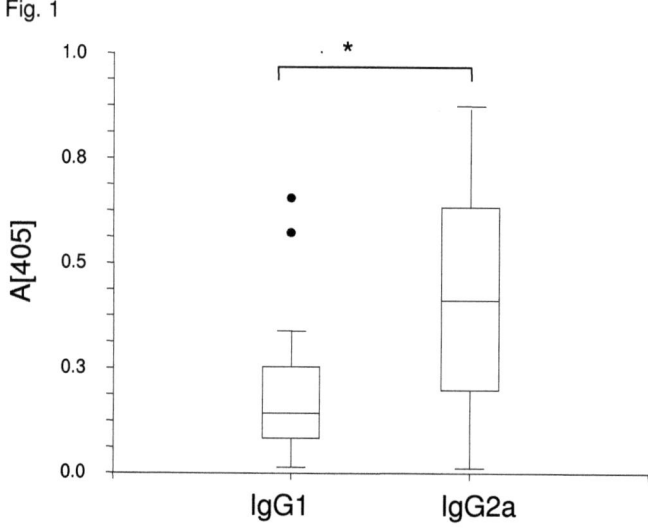

Fig. 2

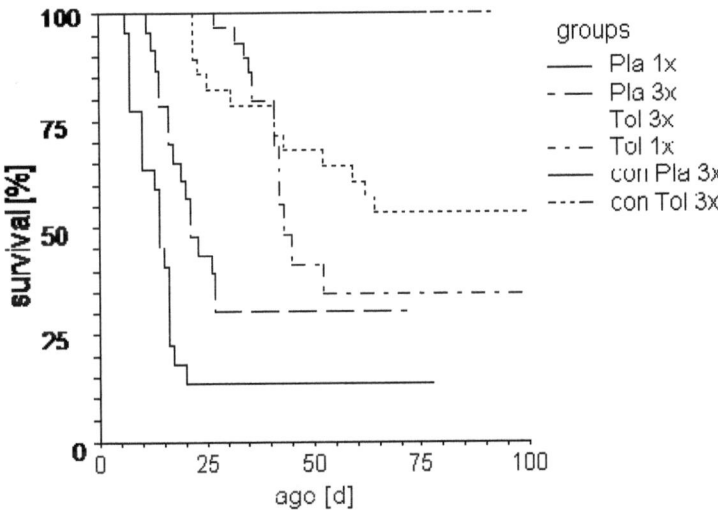

Fig. 3

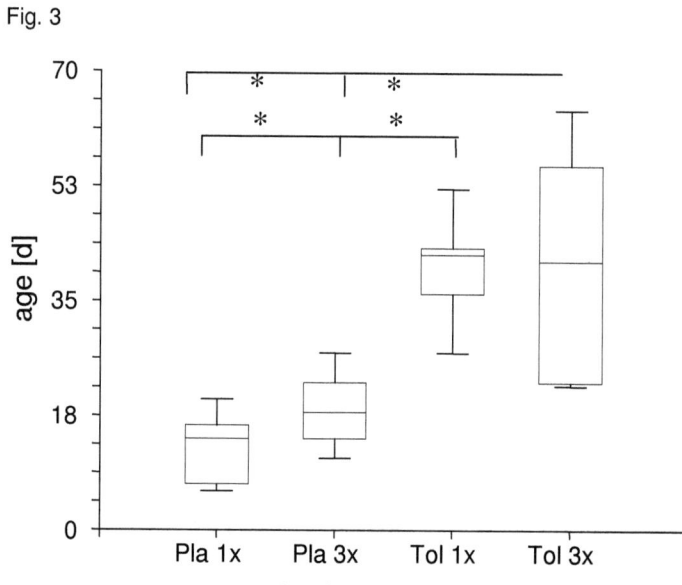

Fig. 4

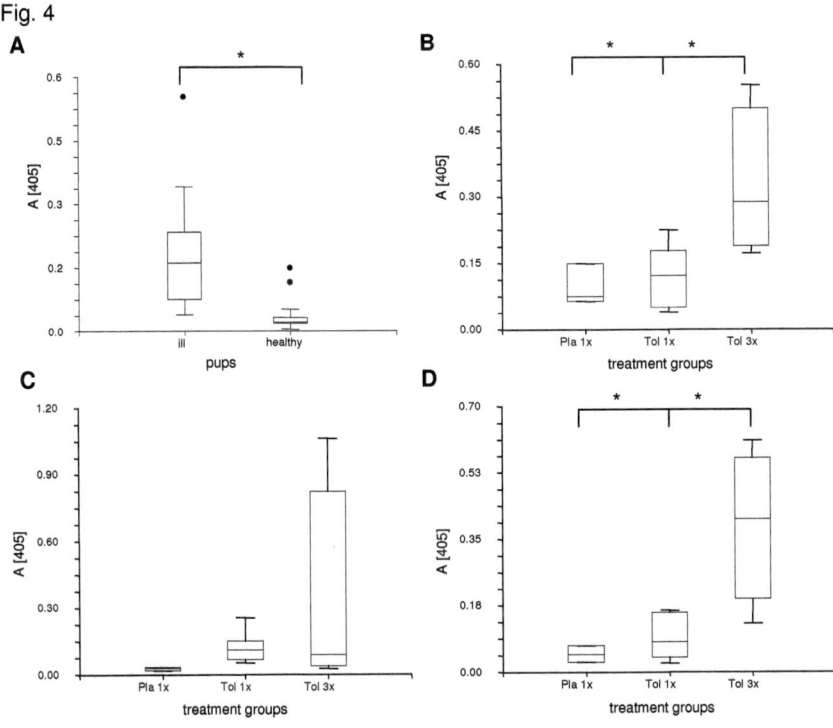

# Survival of *Neospora caninum* inside mouse bone marrow-derived dendritic cells and induction of cytokine expression

Maria Strohbusch[1], Norbert Müller[1], Andrew Hemphill[1], Maxi Margos[1], Denis Grandgirard[2], Gisela Greif[3], Bruno Gottstein[1]*

[1]Institute of Parasitology, University of Bern, Laenggass-Strasse 122, CH-3012 Bern, Switzerland
[2]Institute for Infectious Diseases, University of Bern, Friedbuehlstrasse 51, CH-3010 Bern, Switzerland
[3]Bayer HealthCare AG, Leverkusen, Germany

*address for correspondence:

Institute of Parasitology
Vetsuisse Faculty
University of Bern
Laenggassstrasse 122
CH-3001 Bern, Switzerland
+41 31 631 24 18
bruno.gottstein@ipa.unibe.ch

## Abstract

Dendritic cells (DCs) are the first defence of the innate immune system after infection with pathogens. So far, nothing is known about invasion and survival ability of *Neospora caninum*, a parasite causing abortion in cattle worldwide, in mouse bone marrow DCs (mBMDCs). Furthermore, cytokine expression pattern of DCs after contact with tachyzoites is still unknown. In the present study, mBMDCs were exposed to viable (untreated) and different kinds of inactivated (non-viable) parasites. Invasion and survival ability was determined by NcGRA2-RT-PCR and transmission electron microscopy (TEM). Cytokine expression was evaluated by RT-PCR and cytokine ELISA. TEM of DCs stimulated with untreated viable parasites revealed that *N. caninum* was able to invade cells. Further on, parasites could survive and proliferate within DCs, as also proven by NcGRA2-RT-PCR. On the other hand, non-viability of inactivated parasites was shown by NcGRA2-RT-PCR and no viable parasite structures were found by TEM analysis. Cytokine expression analysis (by RT-PCR and ELISA) exhibited that both, untreated and inactivated parasites, stimulate DCs in a way that they express IL-12p40, IL-10 and TNF-α, whereas IL-4 levels were below detection limit. Expression of both IL-12p40 and IL-10 indicated induction of a mixed Th1/Th2 response.

The work present here was a first approach to determine survival and proliferation ability of *N. caninum* in mBMDCs, and to elucidate cytokine expression patterns of DCs after exposure to viable versus non-viable parasites. The fact that native parasites survive inside DCs is important as DCs are competent immune cells that disseminate through the host body. Thereby, migrating DCs can transport tachyzoites from periphery to organs, as it was described for the related parasite *Toxoplasma gondii*.

## Introduction

Dendritic cells (DCs) are the most potent professional antigen presenting cells (APC). There is a tight correlation between DC maturation and the intracellular exogenous antigen-processing pathway, which is important for cross-presentation. Only early immature DCs can transport ingested antigens from the endocytic compartments into the cytosol and perform cross-presentation [1]. Both mouse classical and plasmacytoid DCs generated from bone marrow as well as lymphoid tissue DCs can direct Th1 or Th2 responses depending on the dose of antigen, the state of maturation of the DCs together with the stimulation of DCs by pathogen-derived products [2]. DCs can directly sense pathogen components via TLRs, and respond to this recognition by up-regulation of surface co-stimulatory molecules, secreting cytokines and chemokines, enhancing antigen presentation, and migrating to secondary lymphoid tissues [3].

Extracts of the apicomplexan parasite *Toxoplasma gondii* were found to activate DCs and to stimulate IL-12 production by DCs [4]. By contrast, active *T. gondii* invasion of immature DC suppresses the ability of these cells to participate in innate immunity and to induce adaptive immune responses [5]. Infection of immature DCs allows the parasites to disseminate from the site of infection within cells undergoing steady-state migration to draining lymphoid organs. It was shown that *T. gondii* induces a state of hypermotility in infected DCs *in vitro* and that parasite-infected DCs promote dissemination of *Toxoplasma in vivo* [6]. This benefits that the parasites can reach the brain and skeletal muscles, where tachyzoites undergo differentiation into the encysted bradyzoite forms to establish chronic infection and ensuring parasite transmission.

The related parasite *Neospora caninum* stimulates antigen presentation on splenic DCs from infected BALB/c mice [7]. Nevertheless, nothing is known so far about the invasion ability of *N. caninum* into DCs and the survival of the parasites in these cells. In the present work we used electron microscopy to identify the interaction between live and dead parasites and DCs. Cytokine expression was determined to answer the question of DCs suppression or activation through the parasite.

## Material and Methods

### Tissue culture media, biochemicals and drugs
If not otherwise stated, all tissue culture media were purchased from Gibco-BRL (Basel, Switzerland) and biochemical reagents were from Sigma (Buchs, Switzerland).

### Tissue culture and parasite purification
Cultures of Vero cells were maintained in RPMI 1640 medium (Gibco-BRL, Basel, Switzerland) supplemented with 5% fetal calf serum (FCS), 4 mM L-glutamine, 100 U/ml penicillin G, 100 µg/ml streptomycin and 0.25 µg/ml amphotericin B at 37°C with 5% $CO_2$. Cultures were trypsinized at least once a week. *N. caninum* (Nc-1 isolate) tachyzoites were maintained in Vero cell monolayer cultures, during which time FCS was replaced with immunoglobulin G-free horse serum. Tachyzoites were harvested when they were still intracellular by trypsinization of infected Vero cells followed by repeated passage through a 25-gauge needle. Host cell debris were removed from the parasites by separation on Sephadex-G25 columns as previously described [8]. The tachyzoites were counted using a Neubauer chamber and parasite numbers were adjusted by adding RPMI medium as appropriate for experimental infection.

### Mice
Wild-type C57BL/6 mice were purchased from Charles River Laboratories (Sulzfeld, Germany) and maintained under conventional day / night-cycle housing conditions as required by the animal welfare legislation of the Swiss Veterinary Office. Food mix and water were provided *ad libitum*. Mice were euthanized by $CO_2$-inhalation.

### Generation and culture of bone marrow dendritic cells (BMDC)
DCs were generated from bone marrow (BM) progenitors as described previously [9]. Briefly, $2 \times 10^6$ bone marrow cells derived from mouse tibia and femur of the hind legs were incubated in petri dishes containing 10 ml RPMI 1640 medium (Gibco-BRL) supplemented with 10% FCS, 2 mM L-glutamine, 100 U/ml penicillin G, 100 µg/ml streptomycin, 0.05 mM β-mercaptoethanol in the presence of 200 U granulocyte-macrophage colony-stimulating factor (GM-CSF; ImmunoTools, Friesoythe, Germany). Cultures were fed with 5 ml fresh supplemented medium

containing 200 U GM-CSF on day 3 and 6. After 9 days, nonadherent cells were collected centrifuged for 10 min at 400 g and viable cells were counted by trypan-blue exclusion using the Neubauer chamber. Cell number was adjusted to $1 \times 10^6$ cells per ml in supplemented medium without GM-CSF and cells were plated in 24 well plates for the corresponding experiments. Preparation contained 75 to 85% $CD11c^+$ cells as determined with FACS analysis (data not shown).

**Stimulation of BMDC and sample collection**

Stimulation of immature DCs was designed as described below:
- (I) $1 \times 10^6$ live Nc-1 tachyzoites
- (II) $1 \times 10^6$ dead Nc-1 tachyzoites (one freezing / thaw cycle in liquid $N_2$)
- (III) $1 \times 10^6$ heat-inactivated Nc-1 tachyzoites (56 °C, 50 min)
- (IV) $1 \times 10^6$ paraformaldehyde (PFA) -inactivated Nc-1 tachyzoites (1.5% paraformaldehyde, 10 min, 5 x wash with medium)
- (V) 100 ng/ml LPS as a positive control
- (VI) medium as a negative control.

To analyse viability of parasites, immature DCs were stimulated as described above and maintained for 0 h, 3 h, 6 h, 18 h, 24 h and 48 h. Cells were directly lysed in the well using 400 µl RTL-buffer (RNeasy® mini kit; QIAGEN, Basel, Switerland) containing 1% β-mercaptoethanol and stored at -80 °C for RNA isolation.

For transmission electron microscopy (TEM) preparation, immature DCs were stimulated as described above. Cells were maintained for 1 h and 48 h and directly prepared for TEM analysis.

For cytokine measurement, immature DCs were stimulated as described above. To control whether parasites suppress cytokine expression of DCs, same stimulants were prepared as described above and LPS (100 ng/ml) was added to samples (I) to (IV). Pre-titration experiments revealed 6 h and 24 h post stimulation as best time points to analyse cytokine expression on mRNA and protein level. Samples for cytokine analysis were taken before (0 h) and 6 h and 24 h after stimulation. Supernatants were collected and stored at -20 °C for cytokine ELISA. Cells were directly lysed in the well using 400 µl RTL-buffer (RNeasy® mini kit; QIAGEN) containing 1% β-mercaptoethanol and stored at -80 °C for RNA isolation.

## RNA extraction

Total RNA isolation from cell cultures was performed using the RNeasy® mini kit (QIAGEN) according to the standard protocol suitable for cells. Frozen lysates were allowed to thaw at 37 °C. All purification steps were performed at room temperature. RNA purification included a DNA digestion step with RNase-free DNase (QIAGEN) for 1 h at room temperature. RNA was eluted in 60 µl RNase-free water, boiled at 95 °C for 3 min and immediately used for cDNA synthesis.

## Reverse Transcription

cDNA synthesis was performed using the Omniscript® Reverse Transcription kit (QIAGEN) according to the standard protocol for first-strand cDNA synthesis. Briefly, 0.5 µg random Primer (Promega, Wallisellen, Switzerland) and 2 µl of RNA were used in a final volume of 20 µl reaction mix and incubated for 1 h at 37 °C. cDNA was boiled at 95 °C for 3 min and frozen at -80 °C prior to PCR.

## Parasite quantification

Quantification of live parasites by real-time RT-PCR was carried out on a LightCycler instrument (Roche Diagnostics; Rotkreuz, Switzerland). NcGRA2-RT-PCR was done as recently described [10] using QuantiTec™SYBR®Green PCR kit (QIAGEN), *N. caninum*-specific primers NcGRA2-F1 and NcGRA2-R2 (10 µM each) and 1:41 diluted cDNA. PCRs were performed with 4.1 µl sample in a final volume of 10 µl. To avoid carry-over contaminations, UDG was added to the mix. As external standards, samples containing cDNA equivalents from 100, 10 and 1 *N. caninum* tachyzoite(s) or only water were included. Parasite number was calculated by assessing mean values (plus standard deviations) from triplicate determinations.

## TEM preparation

TEM sample preparation was done as recently described [11]. Briefly, cells were fixed at 4 °C overnight in 100 mM sodium cacodylate buffer (pH 7.2) containing 2.5% glutaraldehyde, followed by prestaining in 2% $OsO_4$ for 3 h. After washing, pellets were stained for another 1 h in saturated uranyl acetate, followed by extensive washing in water. Dehydration was done in graded series of ethanol (30, 50, 70, 90 and 100%) and dehydrated pellets were embedded in Epon 820 resin for 20 h with two resin changes. The resin was polymerized at 65 °C overnight. Ultrathin sections, loaded onto 300-mesh copper grids, were viewed on a Philips 400 transmission electron microscope.

## Cytokine expression on mRNA level

Amplification of murine gene sequences from β-actin and different cytokines (IL4, IL10, IL12, TNF-α) was performed on a LightCycler instrument (Roche Diagnostics) using QuantiTec™SYBR®Green PCR kit (QIAGEN) and primer pairs designed by Overbergh et al. [12].

| | |
|---|---|
| β-actin-for | AGA GGG AAA TCG TGC GTG AC |
| β-actin-rev | CAA TAG TGA TGA CCT GGC CGT |
| IL4-for | ACA GGA GAA GGG ACG CCA T |
| IL4-rev | GAA GCC CTA CAG ACG AGC TCA |
| IL10-for | GGT TGC CAA GCC TTA TCG GA |
| IL10-rev | ACC TGC TCC ACT GCC TTG CT |
| IL12p40-for | GGA AGC ACG GCA GCA GAA TA |
| IL12p40-rev | AAC TTG AGG GAG AAG TAG GAA TGG |
| TNF-α-for | CAT CTT CTC AAA ATT ATT CGA GTG ACA A |
| TNF-α-rev | TGG GAG TAG ACA AGG TAC AAC CC |

Quantitative PCR was adapted from Bienz et al. [13] using 4 µl of 1:100 diluted cDNA and 0.5 µM of forward and reverse primer in a 10 µl reaction. Mixes were supplemented with $MgCl_2$ to a final concentration of 3 mM. All PCRs containing cDNA were performed in triplicates and one negative control containing water was included in each run. PCR was started by initiating the Hot-Start Taq DNA polymerase reaction at 95 °C (20 min), followed by 50 cycles of DNA amplification (denaturation: 95 °C, 10 sec; annealing: 60 °C, 10 sec; extension: 72 °C, 10 sec). Fluorescence was measured after each cycle at 80 °C. To calculate the slope and the efficacy of the PCR, serial 10-fold dilutions of probes were included for each primer pair and a standard curve was generated. In order to compensate for variation in mRNA amounts, expression of housekeeping gene β-actin was evaluated. Respective mean values from triplicate determinations were taken for calculation of relative cytokine mRNA levels (cytokine mRNA level/β-actin mRNA level) and given in arbitrary units (AU).

## Cytokine ELISA

Cytokine ELISA was performed using the Milliplex™ mouse cytokine kit (Millipore Corporation, Billerica, MA, US) according to the standard protocol for tissue culture supernatant. This technique allows the simultaneous quantification of multiple cytokines using small sample volumes. Following cytokines were assessed: IL-10 (3.3), IL-12p40 (4.9) and TNF-α (1.0). Respective minimal detection limits are shown in brackets (pg/mL). Samples were centrifuged before the assay and studied undiluted in duplets. No detection of IL-4 was done, as already mRNA level of IL-4 was below the detection limit. Fluorescence was measured using Luminex 200 system (Luminex Corp., Austin, TX). Data were analyzed using a five-parametric logistic curve fitting using Bioplex manager software 4.01 (BioRad Laboratories Inc., Hercules, CA).

## Statistical analyses

Significance of the differences between cytokine concentration or mRNA levels of negative control and experimental assays was determined by Student`s $t$ test, using the Microsoft Excel program. Further, differences in the amount of viable parasites between treated and untreated tachyzoites was determined by Student`s $t$ test, using the Microsoft Excel program. $P$ values of <0.05 were considered statistically significant.

## Results

### Viability of *N. caninum*

Viability of untreated and differently inactivated parasites was tested using the NcGRA2-RT-PCR (Fig. 1). Untreated parasites were able to survive within DCs. Furthermore, proliferation was observed from 24 h post infection (pi) on. Treatment with freezing-thawing cycles in liquid nitrogen, heat (56 °C) or 1.5% PFA killed the parasites and no RNA expression was detectable from the beginning until the end of the experiment.

### TEM

Stimulated DCs were used at different time points after adding parasites for TEM preparation. DCs exposed to untreated (viable) tachyzoites contained visible tachyzoites already 1 h pi (Fig. 2A). All common organelles were observed in these tachyzoites without destruction, assuming that parasites were alive. Parasitophorous vacuoles containing proliferating parasites were seen at 48 h pi (Fig. 2B). Although DCs stimulated with 1.5%-PFA-treated parasites contained visible tachyzoites 1 h post infection, these parasites have been found dead (Fig. 2C). PFA-treatment killed parasites, but conserved structures. Empty tachyzoites or tachyzoites containing large vacuoles were observed in DCs stimulated with PFA-treated parasites (Fig. 2C). No visible parasite structures were seen at later time points. Finally, in DCs stimulated with liquid $N_2$- or heat-treated parasites no visible parasite structures were found at 1 h and 48 h pi (data not shown).

### Cytokine expression

DCs and supernatants were collected before stimulation, as well as 6 h and 24 h post stimulation. Cytokine expression analysis on mRNA basis of stimulated DCs revealed expression of IL-10, IL-12p40 and TNF-α mRNA (Fig. 3A-C). IL-4 mRNA levels were below detection limit (data not shown). Significantly higher IL-12p40 expression levels - when compared to non-stimulated control - were observed 6 h and 24 h pi for all stimulants (Fig. 3A). IL-10 expression (Fig. 3B) was significantly higher at time points 6 h and 24 h pi when compared to non-stimulated controls, including DCs that were stimulated with LPS, with untreated or with liquid $N_2$-treated parasites. Heat-treated parasites induced a significant increase of IL-10 expression in DCs after 6 h only, when compared to non-stimulated controls. DCs stimulated with PFA-treated parasites did not show any differences in IL-10 expression when compared to non-stimulated controls. TNF-α expression (Fig. 3C) was significantly increased for both 6 h and 24 h pi, in DCs stimulated with untreated parasites only, when compared to non-stimulated controls. Furthermore, at 24 h pi, TNF-α expression was significant higher when compared to non-stimulated controls in DCs stimulated with LPS or liquid $N_2$-treated parasites. Conversely, stimulation of DCs with PFA-treated parasites resulted in a significant decrease of TNF-α expression at 6 h pi when compared to non-stimulated controls.

Calculation of IL-12p40 concentration (Fig. 4A) in supernatants revealed a significant increase of this cytokine 24 h pi for all stimulants when compared to non-stimulated controls. Only stimulation with LPS, liquid $N_2$- and heat-treated parasites induced significantly higher IL-12p40 concentrations at 6 h pi already, when compared to non-stimulated controls. IL-10 concentration (Fig. 4B) was significantly increased at 6 h and 24 h after stimulation of DCs with LPS, untreated and heat-treated parasites, when compared to non-stimulated controls, whereas liquid $N_2$-treated parasites significantly increased IL-10 concentrations at 6 h pi, and PFA-treated parasites at 24 h pi only. Compared to non-stimulated controls, TNF-α concentration (Fig. 4C) was significantly higher at 6 h and 24 h pi for all stimulants.

To prove whether *N. caninum* has any direct inhibitory effect on cytokine expression, LPS was added to DCs stimulated with untreated and inactivated and parasites. No inhibitory effect was observed, as addition of LPS resulted in increasing cytokine mRNA levels and concentrations for all kinds of parasite preparations (data not shown).

## Discussion

Dendritic cells are the most potent professional antigen presenting cells and specialized to activate innate and adaptive immune responses. Both mouse classical and plasmacytoid DCs can direct Th1 or Th2 responses [2]. Apicomplexan parasites, like *T. gondii*, were found to activate DCs and to stimulate IL-12 production by DCs [4].

In the present work, interaction of *N. caninum* with immature mBMDCs was evaluated for the first time. It was shown that viable parasites invaded DCs, survived and started to proliferate inside these cells. DCs are competent immune cells that disseminate through the host body. Thereby, migrating DCs can transport live tachyzoites from periphery to organs, as it was described for the related parasite *T. gondii* [6]. The fact that *N. caninum* survived in DCs *in vitro* leads to presume that parasites use this possibility to disseminate between different organs and last but not least, to reach the brain. Further on, untreated and therefore viable parasites stimulated DCs to produce cytokines, like IL-12p40, IL-10 and TNF-α, at significantly higher levels than non-stimulated cells. TNF-α is involved in systemic inflammation and is a member of a group of cytokines that all stimulate acute phase reactions. Large amounts of TNF-α are released in response to LPS. IL-12 is a major inducer of Th1 responses, whereas IL-10 induces Th2 responses. Dependent on the dose of the antigen, DCs can lead to Th1, Th2 or mixed Th1/Th2 responses, whereas high antigen doses induce Th1 and low antigen doses Th2 responses [2]. Infection of DCs with one parasite per cell induced both IL-12p40 and IL-10 expression, causing a mixed Th1/Th2 response.

On the other hand, inactivated and destroyed parasites were captured through phagocytosis by DCs. Parasites treated with freeze/thaw cycles in liquid $N_2$ were completely destroyed and non-viability was observed right after treatment. Furthermore, no parasite-like structures were detectable in DCs 1 h pi. Nevertheless, parasite extract was taken up by DCs and induced cytokine production already 6 h after stimulation. Again, IL-12p40, IL-10 and TNF-α were verified, leading to a mixed Th1/Th2 response. Although heat inactivation did not destroy parasites, it killed them and non-viability was proven right after treatment. However, no parasite-like structures could be observed inside DCs 1 h after stimulation. Dead parasites were captured by the cells and immediately degraded. Like parasite extract, heat-inactivated parasites led to a mixed Th1/Th2 response. PFA treatment killed parasites, but it also conserved morphological structures. Although parasites were found inside DCs 1 h pi, non-viability of these parasites was proven by NcGRA2-RT-PCR. TEM analysis of PFA-treated parasites inside DCs indicated whole tachyzoites, but with degraded organelles. As this tachyzoite were dead, they had to be taken up by DCs through phagocytosis. However, PFA-treated parasites were completely processed by DCs and no parasite-like structures were visible at later time points. Furthermore, PFA-treated parasites induced a Th1/Th2 phenotype of DCs.

In this study, it was shown for the first time that *N. caninum* invaded immature mBMDCs and was able to proliferate in these cells. Furthermore, stimulation with one live or inactivated parasite per DC led to a mixed Th1/Th2 response, marked by expression of IL-12p40 and IL-10. These DCs can be a useful tool to induce distinct T-cell responses. In addition, DCs stimulated with live parasites can provide more information about parasite dissemination within the host.

## References

[1.] Hotta C, Fujimaki H, Yoshinari M, Nakazawa M, Minami M. The delivery of an antigen from the endocytic compartment into the cytosol for cross-presentation is restricted to early immature dendritic cells. Immunology 2006;117(1):97-107.

[2.] Boonstra A, Asselin-Paturel C, Gilliet M, Crain C, Trinchieri G, Liu YJ, O'Garra A. Flexibility of mouse classical and plasmacytoid-derived dendritic cells in directing T helper type 1 and 2 cell development: dependency on antigen dose and differential toll-like receptor ligation. J Exp Med 2003;197(1):101-9.

[3.] Iwasaki A, Medzhitov R. Toll-like receptor control of the adaptive immune responses. Nat Immunol 2004;5(10):987-95.

[4.] Reis e Sousa C, Hieny S, Scharton-Kersten T, Jankovic D, Charest H, Germain RN, Sher A. In vivo microbial stimulation induces rapid CD40 ligand-independent production of interleukin 12 by dendritic cells and their redistribution to T cell areas. J Exp Med 1997;186(11):1819-29.

[5.] McKee AS, Dzierszinski F, Boes M, Roos DS, Pearce EJ. Functional inactivation of immature dendritic cells by the intracellular parasite *Toxoplasma gondii*. J Immunol 2004;173(4):2632-40.

[6.] Lambert H, Hitziger N, Dellacasa I, Svensson M, Barragan A. Induction of dendritic cell migration upon *Toxoplasma gondii* infection potentiates parasite dissemination. Cell Microbiol 2006;8(10):1611-23.

[7.] Veeraseatakul P, Chutipongvivate S. Major histocompatibility complex class II and co-stimulatory molecule CD80 expression in splenic dendritic cells from BALB/c mice infected with *Neospora caninum*. J Trop Med Parasitol 2005;28:31-8.

[8.] Hemphill A, Gottstein B, Kaufmann H. Adhesion and invasion of bovine endothelial cells by *Neospora caninum*. Parasitology 1996;112 (Pt 2):183-97.

[9.] Lutz MB, Kukutsch N, Ogilvie AL, Rossner S, Koch F, Romani N, Schuler G. An advanced culture method for generating large quantities of highly pure dendritic cells from mouse bone marrow. J Immunol Methods 1999;223(1):77-92.

[10.] Strohbusch M, Müller N, Hemphill A, Greif G, Gottstein B. NcGRA2 as a molecular target to assess the parasiticidal activity of toltrazuril against *Neospora caninum*. Parasitology 2008;135(9):1065-73.

[11.] Leepin A, Stüdli A, Brun R, Stephens CE, Boykin DW, Hemphill A. Host cells participate in the in vitro effects of novel diamidine analogues against tachyzoites of the intracellular apicomplexan parasites *Neospora caninum* and *Toxoplasma gondii*. Antimicrob Agents Chemother 2008;52(6):1999-2008.

[12.] Overbergh L, Valckx D, Waer M, Mathieu C. Quantification of murine cytokine mRNAs using real time quantitative reverse transcriptase PCR. Cytokine 1999;11(4):305-12.

[13.] Bienz M, Dai WJ, Welle M, Gottstein B, Müller N. Interleukin-6-deficient mice are highly susceptible to *Giardia lamblia* infection but exhibit normal intestinal immunoglobulin A responses against the parasite. Infect Immun 2003;71(3):1569-73.

**Figure legends**

**Figure 1**

Viability of *N. caninum* inside DCs. Viability was proven with NcGRA2-RT-PCR at 3 h, 6 h, 18 h, 24 h and 48 h after infection of DCs. Parasites were treated with freeze/thaw cycles in liquid $N_2$ (■), 56 °C for 50 min (▲), 1.5% PFA (●) or lead untreated (♦). 0 h presents time point after treatment, but before adding to DCs. Different treatment techniques killed parasites, as no viability could be observed right after treatment until the end of the experiment. On the other hand, untreated parasites were alive over the whole time period. Actually, tachyzoites were able to proliferate inside DCs after 24 h. Amount of viable parasites in the untreated group was significant higher than in the treated group (* $P < 0.05$).

**Figure 2**

TEM analysis. DCs stimulated with treated and untreated parasites were used at 1 h and 48 h pi for TEM preparation. (A) Untreated tachyzoite inside DC 1 h after infection. Common organelles were visible and not destroyed. (B) Untreated tachyzoites inside DCs 48 h after infection. Parasitophorous vacuole with proliferating parasites (arrow) was observed. (C) PFA-treated (1.5% PFA) tachyzoite inside DCs 1 h after infection. Only parasite form was identifiable, whereas organelles were almost destroyed. C: conoid, D: dense granule, DC: dendritic cell, G: golgi body, M: micronemes, n: nucleus of DC, N: nucleus of parasite, R: rhoptries, T: tachyzoite.

**Figure 3**

Cytokine expression on mRNA level. IL-12p40 (A), IL-10 (B) and TNF-α mRNA levels of DCs stimulated with LPS, viable and inactivated parasites were determined before (0 h) and 6 h and 24 h after stimulation. mRNA levels were described relative to the housekeeping gene β-actin as arbitrary units (AU). Significant ($P < 0.05$) increase or decrease of expression relative to the non-stimulated control (neg) was calculated and significance after 6 h stimulation was labelled with * and after 24 h with [&]. live Nc-1: untreated parasites, N2: parasites treated with freeze/thaw cycles in liquid nitrogen, heat: parasite inactivation at 56°C, PFA: parasites treated with 1.5% PFA.

**Figure 4**

Cytokine ELSIA to measure cytokine concentration. IL-12p40 (A), IL-10 (B) and TNF-α concentration in supernatants from DCs stimulated with LPS, viable and inactivated parasites were determined before (0 h) and 6 h and 24 h after stimulation. Significant ($P < 0.05$) increase of cytokine concentration relative to the non-stimulated control (neg) was calculated and significance after 6 h stimulation was labelled with * and after 24 h with [&]. live Nc-1: untreated parasites, N2: parasites treated with freeze/thaw cycles in liquid nitrogen, heat: parasite inactivation at 56°C, PFA: parasites treated with 1.5% PFA.

Fig. 1

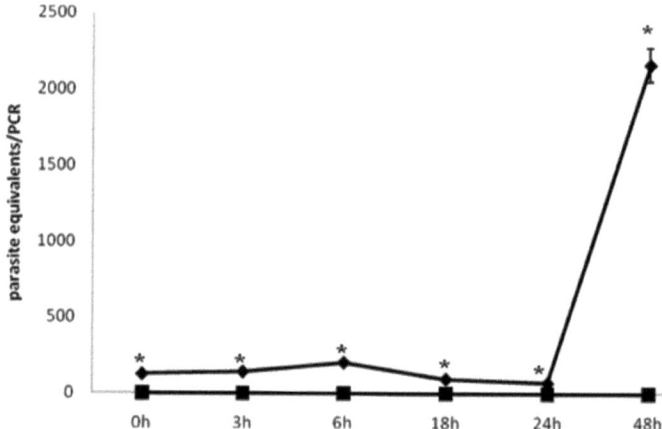

Fig. 2

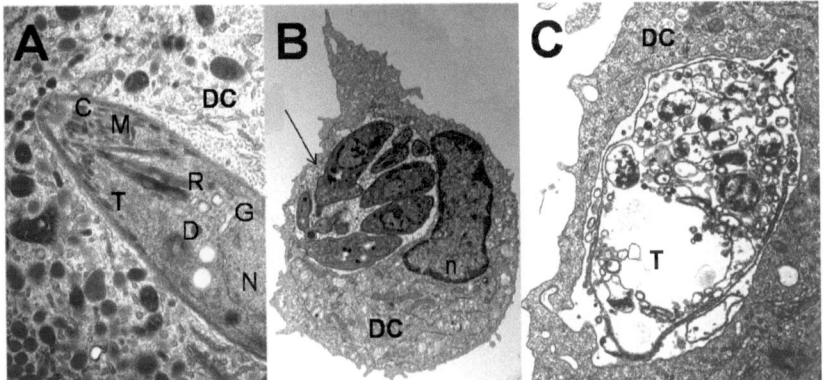

Fig. 3

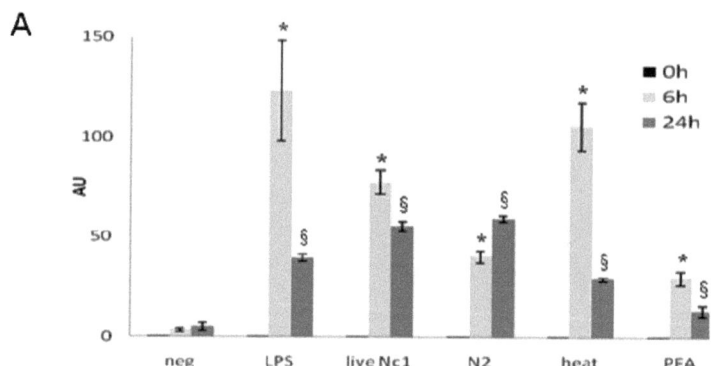
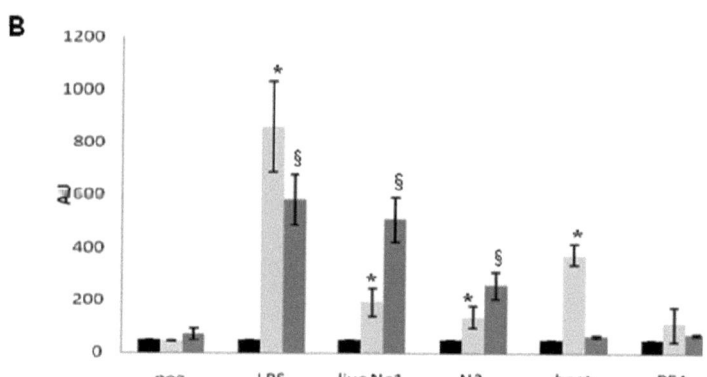
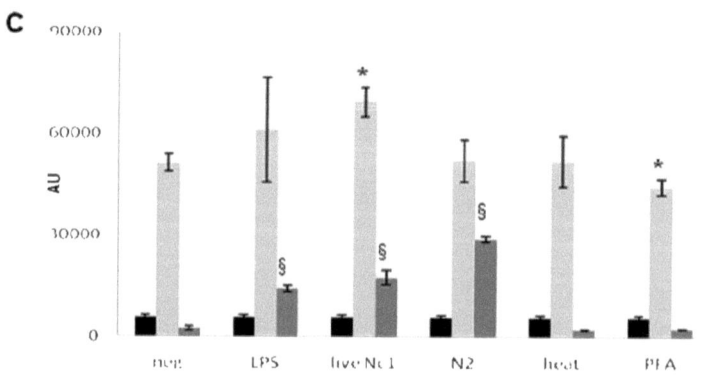

Fig. 4

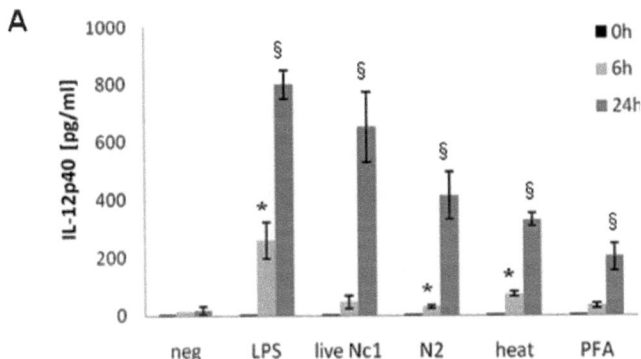

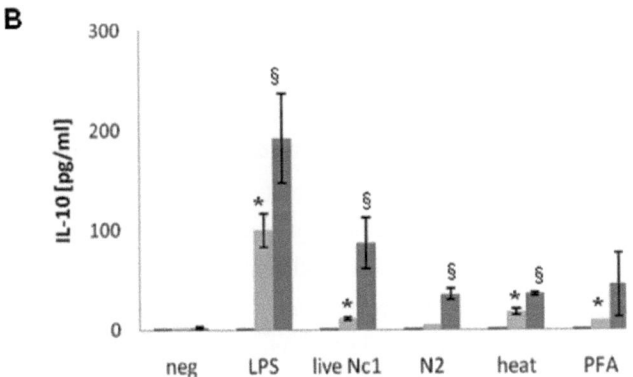

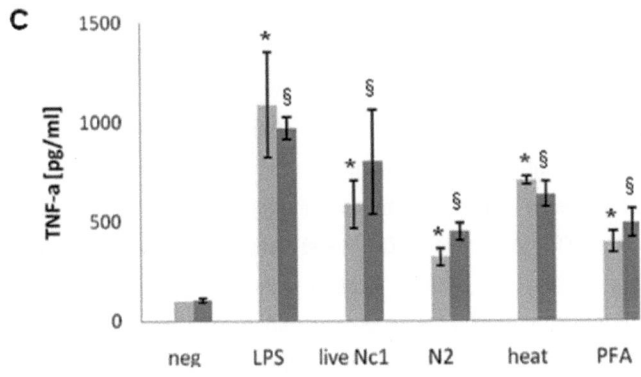

# Discussion

Current evidence strongly indicates that *Neospora caninum* is the protozoan pathogen most commonly associated with bovine abortion worldwide, causing serious veterinary health and economic problems within livestock production (Dubey et al., 2007). So far, there is no treatment available to remove the parasite from an infected herd and the only way to get rid of an infection is culling of infected animals. A wide range of compounds have been tested in cell culture-based assays and in experimentally infected mice and cattle. Toltrazuril, a symmetric trazinone derivative, was found to exhibit anti-coccidial activity against cyst-forming and non-cyst-forming coccidian parasites. The drug was successfully tested in cell culture-based assays and in the mouse model against *N. caninum* infections.

The present study represents a further step in assessing the efficacy of toltrazuril against *N. caninum* infections in both, cell culture and mouse model. With cell culture-based assays, the anti-parasitic effect of toltrazuil was determined. The results indicated a parasitostatic activity after short term treatment of at least two days. A parasiticidal activity of toltrazuril was first observed after a 14-day-treatment period. The fact that at least 14 days of *in vitro* treatment were necessary to obtain parasiticidal activity, has important implications for the development of novel treatment strategies. The data were used to provide baseline information about the effects of repeated toltrazuril treatments on congenitally *N. caninum*-infected newborn mice, prior to carrying out similar future experiments in the bovine system. The results of the present study indicated that the treatment with three application of toltrazuril right after birth had best positive effects for controlling the course of infection in congenitally *N. caninum*-infected newborn mice. No negative side-effects were observed after three high doses of toltrazuril in uninfected mice. Newborn mice were as effective as adults in developing primary antigen-specific T-cell population within the first week of life (Adkins and Du, 1998) and were thus fully immune competent at this age (Morein et al., 2002). Applied to the present experiments, this allows the conclusion that congenitally infected pups appeared to have mounted a T-cell-immune response effectively supporting the toltrazuril treatment. In order to provide an appropriate and constant high toltrazuril concentration in mice for at least 14 days, repeated applications of toltrazuril seemed to be necessary. The advantage of treating congenitally infected neonates is – in case of success - the longterm production of defined parasite-free animal stocks which can be used to create parasite-free breeding lines. If other risk factors for a re-infection can be excluded, the prevalence of infection and disease within a herd could be reduced or even abrogated. Toltrazuril is already used in veterinary medicine to treat coccidiosis of poultry and certain mammalian animal species. From this point of view, it would be no problem to adapt the treatment schedule to eliminate also possible *N. caninum* infections. Calves from infected cows will mostly be born without clinical signs of neosporosis and detection of *Neospora* antibodies does not necessarily imply that these calves are infected. Preventive treatment with toltrazuril without negative side-effects would be a useful and safe strategy to eliminate parasites from the herd without culling animals. Because of the lower body weight of newborns, a lower amount of drug is needed (in comparison to adult animals), which would also lower the costs. Furthermore, withdrawal time with respect to meat and milk production would not be a problem.

There are a number of different diagnostic tools available to detect *N. caninum* and to discriminate neosporosis from infections with closely related parasites. However, the presence of parasite gDNA or antigens in infected tissue does not necessarily provide information on parasite viability, and conventional *in vivo* and *in vitro* tests are being used by inoculating appropriate samples into laboratory animals or cell culture (Dubey et al., 2007). These methods can often be time-consuming and inconclusive. The distinction between live and dead organism is an important tool, for example, in testing of chemotherapeutical compounds or for vaccination studies. In the present study, a RT-PCR based on the *NcGRA2* gene was established to distinguish between live and dead parasites, making use of specific RNA available in live organisms. Although *NcGRA2* shares 56% sequence homology with the *Toxoplasma GRA2* (Ellis et al., 2000), the NcGRA2-RT-PCR is specific for *Neospora*. The NcGRA2-RT-PCR was validated with regards to short-term and long-term effects of toltrazuril in cell culture. With the novel test, parasitostatic activity of toltrazuril was observed after short-term treatment, whereas parasiticidal efficacy needed 14 days of treatment. These findings are important to develop therapeutic treatment strategies. The NcGRA2-RT-PCR was also adapted to detect live parasites in organs from *Neospora*-infected mice. In comparison with an alternative inoculation of material in cell culture, the NcGRA2-RT-PCR was much faster and easier to handle. Further, there was less risk of sample contamination if PCR was done with material freshly isolated from mouse tissue instead of culturing material for 4 weeks.

In the present thesis, it was reported for the first time that *N. caninum* is able to invade immature mouse bone marrow-derived dendritic cells (mBMDCs), to survive and even to proliferate within these immune competent cells. This fact leads to the discussion whether *N. caninum* uses DCs to disseminate within the host body. Within migrating DCs, parasites could reach muscles and brain tissue, bypassing host immune system. Inside muscles and brain tissue tachyzoites transform into bradyzoites, which are resistant against immune factors and can persist within the host for several years. Interestingly, not only inactivated parasites and parasites extract, but also live parasites, induced cytokine expression in DCs. Stimulation with both, live and dead parasites, resulted in a mixed Th1/Th2 response characterized by expression of IL-12p40 and IL-10.

# Perspectives

Prevalence of N. caninum in cattle ranges between 1 and 80% worldwide (as assessed upon serological means). So far, the only available vaccination (Bovilis® Neoguard, Intervet) yielded very controversial findings and has thus not been propagated in many European countries. Therefore, chemotherapeutical medication is a highly proposed aim and quite a lot of compounds were tested in cell culture and experimentally infected animals. In the thesis presented here, the triazinone derivative toltrazuril was further characterized with regards to parasitostatic versus parasiticidal activity in cell culture and with regard to the effect on congenitally acquired N. caninum infection in newborn mice. As mice and cell culture-based assays are only experimental models, the main aim is to carry out definitive experiments in the bovine target species. Results obtained from the small animal model and cell culture-based assays can be used to design experiments in cattle without wasting time and animals.

The results provided in this thesis will be useful for planning future medication studies to treat congenitally infected calves. Treatment has to be designed in a way that the toltrazuril plasma levels remain high enough for at last 14 days in order to achieve parasiticidal activity. Treatment of congenitally infected calves has the potential to eliminate N. caninum before tissue cysts have been developed. However, in order to reach optimal efficacy, toltrazuril will also have to be tested against tissue cysts including bradyzoites. To examine this, the already available *in vitro* production of bradyzoites has to be improved to obtain nearly 100% bradyzoites. After determination of the best *in vitro* treatment strategy, application can be adapted for treating tissue cysts in small animal models and later also in cattle. Further interesting questions are: (I) in which amount the drug can cross the blood-brain-barrier; and (II) in which concentration toltrazuril can accumulate within the brain. Drug concentration and duration of activity in the brain are important parameters that have to be validated to be sure that toltrazuril is available for at least 14 days in adequate concentrations for achieving parasiticidal activity. Presently, these parameters were evaluated in the mouse model. As soon as the effective concentration of toltrazuril in serum and brain at different time points after treatment is known, treatment schedules can be optimized and adapted to produce constant drug concentrations over the respective time period.

A useful tool to distinguish between live and dead parasites during and after vaccination and treatment studies is the NcGRA2-RT-PCR. This PCR is specific for detection of live *N. caninum* tachyzoites and should also work for bradyzoites, as the NcGRA2 protein was found in bradyzoites. To confirm this, again, clearly defined bradyzoites will have to be produced without any contamination of tachyzoites. Further, nothing is known about the expression of NcGRA2 in sporozoites. To demonstrate this, live and dead sporozoites will have to be tested with the new RT-PCR.

Another important application for the NcGRA2-RT-PCR is to identify live parasites in tissue of infected animals instead of inoculating material in immunocompremised animals. Adaptation of the RT-PCR to achieve identical or similar sensitivities as reached in immunocompremised aninmal assays would reduce waste of animals, but would also be faster, cheaper and easier to handle.

So far, nothing is known about the interaction of *N. caninum* with immune competent cells, like dendritic cells. In the present work, it was shown that *N. caninum* was able to survive and proliferate within DCs. Examination of parasite strategies used to avoid DC digestion would provide an important insight into parasite survival within the host immune defence. An interesting approach would be to find out whether *Neospora* is able to modify DCs in a way that parasites could use DCs to migrate and disseminate through the host body. Another interesting point to adress is, how *Neospora*-infected DCs influence the host immune system. This in view to use *in vitro* stimulated DCs as vaccine candidates. To get a first overview, mixed leucocyte reactions can be performed using *Neospora*-infected DCs to stimulated naïve T-cells. Futhermore, immature DCs should be stimulated with different parasite concentrations, as different antigen dosing can direct DCs to produce Th1- or Th2- stimulating cytokines.

# References

Adkins, B., 2005, Neonatal T cell function. J Pediatr Gastroenterol Nutr 40 Suppl 1, S5-7.
Adkins, B., Du, R.Q., 1998, Newborn mice develop balanced Th1/Th2 primary effector responses *in vivo* but are biased to Th2 secondary responses. J Immunol 160, 4217-4224.
Alaeddine, F., Keller, N., Leepin, A., Hemphill, A., 2005, Reduced infection and protection from clinical signs of cerebral neosporosis in C57BL/6 mice vaccinated with recombinant microneme antigen NcMIC1. J Parasitol 91, 657-665.
Ammann, P., Waldvogel, A., Breyer, I., Esposito, M., Müller, N., Gottstein, B., 2004, The role of B- and T-cell immunity in toltrazuril-treated C57BL/6 WT, microMT and nude mice experimentally infected with *Neospora caninum*. Parasitol Res 93, 178-187.
Andrianarivo, A.G., Barr, B.C., Anderson, M.L., Rowe, J.D., Packham, A.E., Sverlow, K.W., Conrad, P.A., 2001, Immune responses in pregnant cattle and bovine fetuses following experimental infection with *Neospora caninum*. Parasitol Res 87, 817-825.
Antony, A., Williamson, N.B., 2003, Prevalence of antibodies to *Neospora caninum* in dogs of rural or urban origin in central New Zealand. N Z Vet J 51, 232-237.
Barber, J.S., Gasser, R.B., Ellis, J., Reichel, M.P., McMillan, D., Trees, A.J., 1997, Prevalence of antibodies to *Neospora caninum* in different canid populations. J Parasitol 83, 1056-1058.
Barber, J.S., Trees, A.J., 1996, Clinical aspects of 27 cases of neosporosis in dogs. Vet Rec 139, 439-443.
Barr, B.C., Conrad, P.A., Sverlow, K.W., Tarantal, A.F., Hendrickx, A.G., 1994, Experimental fetal and transplacental *Neospora* infection in the nonhuman primate. Lab Invest 71, 236-242.
Bartels, C.J., Arnaiz-Seco, J.I., Ruiz-Santa-Quitera, A., Björkman, C., Frossling, J., von Blumroder, D., Conraths, F.J., Schares, G., van Maanen, C., Wouda, W., Ortega-Mora, L.M., 2006, Supranational comparison of *Neospora caninum* seroprevalences in cattle in Germany, The Netherlands, Spain and Sweden. Vet Parasitol 137, 17-27.
Bartley, P.M., Kirvar, E., Wright, S., Swales, C., Esteban-Redondo, I., Buxton, D., Maley, S.W., Schock, A., Rae, A.G., Hamilton, C., Innes, E.A., 2004, Maternal and fetal immune responses of cattle inoculated with *Neospora caninum* at mid-gestation. J Comp Pathol 130, 81-91.
Baszler, T.V., Long, M.T., McElwain, T.F., Mathison, B.A., 1999, Interferon-gamma and interleukin-12 mediate protection to acute *Neospora caninum* infection in BALB/c mice. Int J Parasitol 29, 1635-1646.
Belkaid, Y., Oldenhove, G., 2008, Tuning microenvironments: induction of regulatory T cells by dendritic cells. Immunity 29, 362-371.

Bjerkas, I., Mohn, S.F., Presthus, J., 1984, Unidentified cyst-forming sporozoon causing encephalomyelitis and myositis in dogs. Z Parasitenkd 70, 271-274.

Björkman, Lunden, A., Uggla, A., 1994, Prevalence of antibodies to *Neospora caninum* and *Toxoplasma gondii* in Swedish dogs. Acta Vet Scand 35, 445-447.

Björkman, C., Johansson, O., Stenlund, S., Holmdahl, O.J., Uggla, A., 1996, *Neospora* species infection in a herd of dairy cattle. J Am Vet Med Assoc 208, 1441-1444.

Björkman, C., Naslund, K., Stenlund, S., Maley, S.W., Buxton, D., Uggla, A., 1999, An IgG avidity ELISA to discriminate between recent and chronic *Neospora caninum* infection. J Vet Diagn Invest 11, 41-44.

Boonstra, A., Asselin-Paturel, C., Gilliet, M., Crain, C., Trinchieri, G., Liu, Y.J., O'Garra, A., 2003, Flexibility of mouse classical and plasmacytoid-derived dendritic cells in directing T helper type 1 and 2 cell development: dependency on antigen dose and differential toll-like receptor ligation. J Exp Med 197, 101-109.

Boysen, P., Klevar, S., Olsen, I., Storset, A.K., 2006, The protozoan *Neospora caninum* directly triggers bovine NK cells to produce gamma interferon and to kill infected fibroblasts. Infect Immun 74, 953-960.

Buxton, D., Maley, S.W., Pastoret, P.P., Brochier, B., Innes, E.A., 1997, Examination of red foxes (*Vulpes vulpes*) from Belgium for antibody to *Neospora caninum* and *Toxoplasma gondii.* Vet Rec 141, 308-309.

Buxton, D., McAllister, M.M., Dubey, J.P., 2002, The comparative pathogenesis of neosporosis. Trends Parasitol 18, 546-552.

Cannas, A., Naguleswaran, A., Müller, N., Gottstein, B., Hemphill, A., 2003, Reduced cerebral infection of *Neospora caninum*-infected mice after vaccination with recombinant microneme protein NcMIC3 and ribi adjuvant. J Parasitol 89, 44-50.

Chi, J., VanLeeuwen, J.A., Weersink, A., Keefe, G.P., 2002, Direct production losses and treatment costs from bovine viral diarrhoea virus, bovine leukosis virus, *Mycobacterium avium* subspecies paratuberculosis, and *Neospora caninum*. Prev Vet Med 55, 137-153.

Collantes-Fernàndez, E., Alvarez-Garcia, G., Perez-Perez, V., Pereira-Bueno, J., Ortega-Mora, L.M., 2004, Characterization of pathology and parasite load in outbred and inbred mouse models of chronic *Neospora caninum* infection. J Parasitol 90, 579-583.

Collantes-Fernàndez, E., Lopez-Perez, I., Alvarez-Garcia, G., Ortega-Mora, L.M., 2006, Temporal distribution and parasite load kinetics in blood and tissues during *Neospora caninum* infection in mice. Infect Immun 74, 2491-2494.

Collantes-Fernàndez, E., Zaballos, A., Alvarez-Garcia, G., Ortega-Mora, L.M., 2002, Quantitative detection of *Neospora caninum* in bovine aborted fetuses and experimentally infected mice by real-time PCR. J Clin Microbiol 40, 1194-1198.

Costa, K.S., Santos, S.L., Uzeda, R.S., Pinheiro, A.M., Almeida, M.A., Araujo, F.R., McAllister, M.M., Gondim, L.F., 2008, Chickens (*Gallus domesticus*) are natural intermediate hosts of *Neospora caninum*. Int J Parasitol 38, 157-159.

Damriyasa, I.M., Bauer, C., Edelhofer, R., Failing, K., Lind, P., Petersen, E., Schares, G., Tenter, A.M., Volmer, R., Zahner, H., 2004, Cross-sectional survey in pig breeding farms in Hesse, Germany: seroprevalence and risk factors of infections with *Toxoplasma gondii*, *Sarcocystis* spp. and *Neospora caninum* in sows. Vet Parasitol 126, 271-286.

Darius, A.K., Mehlhorn, H., Heydorn, A.O., 2004, Effects of toltrazuril and ponazuril on *Hammondia heydorni* (syn. *Neospora caninum*) infections in mice. Parasitol Res 92, 520-522.

Darius, A.K., Mehlhorn, H., Heydorn, A.O., 2004, Effects of toltrazuril and ponazuril on the fine structure and multiplication of tachyzoites of the NC-1 strain of *Neospora caninum* (a synonym of *Hammondia heydorni*) in cell cultures. Parasitol Res 92, 453-458.

Debache, K., Guionaud, C., Alaeddine, F., Mevissen, M., Hemphill, A., 2008, Vaccination of mice with recombinant NcROP2 antigen reduces mortality and cerebral infection in mice infected with *Neospora caninum* tachyzoites. Int J Parasitol 38, 1455-1463

Dubey, J.P., 1999, Neosporosis - the first decade of research. Int J Parasitol 29, 1485-1488.

Dubey, J.P., 2003, Review of *Neospora caninum* and neosporosis in animals. Korean J Parasitol 41, 1-16.

Dubey, J.P., Barr, B.C., Barta, J.R., Bjerkas, I., Björkman, C., Blagburn, B.L., Bowman, D.D., Buxton, D., Ellis, J.T., Gottstein, B., Hemphill, A., Hill, D.E., Howe, D.K., Jenkins, M.C., Kobayashi, Y., Koudela, B., Marsh, A.E., Mattsson, J.G., McAllister, M.M., Modry, D., Omata, Y., Sibley, L.D., Speer, C.A., Trees, A.J., Uggla, A., Upton, S.J., Williams, D.J., Lindsay, D.S., 2002, Redescription of Neospora caninum and its differentiation from related coccidia. Int J Parasitol 32, 929-946.

Dubey, J.P., Buxton, D., Wouda, W., 2006, Pathogenesis of bovine neosporosis. J Comp Pathol 134, 267-289.

Dubey, J.P., Carpenter, J.L., Speer, C.A., Topper, M.J., Uggla, A., 1988, Newly recognized fatal protozoan disease of dogs. J Am Vet Med Assoc 192, 1269-1285.

Dubey, J.P., Dorough, K.R., Jenkins, M.C., Liddell, S., Speer, C.A., Kwok, O.C., Shen, S.K., 1998, Canine neosporosis: clinical signs, diagnosis, treatment and isolation of *Neospora caninum* in mice and cell culture. Int J Parasitol 28, 1293-1304.

Dubey, J.P., Hattel, A.L., Lindsay, D.S., Topper, M.J., 1988, Neonatal *Neospora caninum* infection in dogs: isolation of the causative agent and experimental transmission. J Am Vet Med Assoc 193, 1259-1263.

Dubey, J.P., Koestner, A., Piper, R.C., 1990, Repeated transplacental transmission of *Neospora caninum* in dogs. J Am Vet Med Assoc 197, 857-860.

Dubey, J.P., Lindsay, D.S., 1989, Transplacental *Neospora caninum* infection in dogs. Am J Vet Res 50, 1578-1579.
Dubey, J.P., Lindsay, D.S., 1996, A review of *Neospora caninum* and neosporosis. Vet Parasitol 67, 1-59.
Dubey, J.P., Lindsay, D.S., 2000, Gerbils (*Meriones unguiculatus*) are highly susceptible to oral infection with *Neospora caninum* oocysts. Parasitol Res 86, 165-168.
Dubey, J.P., Morales, J.A., Villalobos, P., Lindsay, D.S., Blagburn, B.L., Topper, M.J., 1996, Neosporosis-associated abortion in a dairy goat. J Am Vet Med Assoc 208, 263-265.
Dubey, J.P., Schares, G., Ortega-Mora, L.M., 2007, Epidemiology and control of neosporosis and *Neospora caninum*. Clin Microbiol Rev 20, 323-367.
Dubey, J.P., Zarnke, R., Thomas, N.J., Wong, S.K., Van Bonn, W., Briggs, M., Davis, J.W., Ewing, R., Mense, M., Kwok, O.C., Romand, S., Thulliez, P., 2003, *Toxoplasma gondii*, *Neospora caninum*, *Sarcocystis neurona*, and *Sarcocystis canis*-like infections in marine mammals. Vet Parasitol 116, 275-296.
Ellis, J., Luton, K., Baverstock, P.R., Brindley, P.J., Nimmo, K.A., Johnson, A.M., 1994, The phylogeny of *Neospora caninum*. Mol Biochem Parasitol 64, 303-311.
Ellis, J.T., Ryce, C., Atkinson, R., Balu, S., Jones, P., Harper, P.A., 2000, Isolation, characterization and expression of a GRA2 homologue from *Neospora caninum*. Parasitology 120 (Pt 4), 383-390.
Eperon, S., Brönnimann, K., Hemphill, A., Gottstein, B., 1999, Susceptibility of B-cell deficient C57BL/6 (microMT) mice to *Neospora caninum* infection. Parasite Immunol 21, 225-236.
Esposito, M., Moores, S.L., Hemphill, A., 2006, Nitazoxanide and thiazolides, a novel class of broadspectrum anti-parasitic drugs. Res Adv in Antimicrobial Agents and Chemother 6, 1-11.
Esposito, M., Müller, N., Hemphill, A., 2007, Structure-activity relationships from in vitro efficacies of the thiazolide series against the intracellular apicomplexan protozoan *Neospora caninum*. Int J Parasitol 37, 183-190.
Esposito, M., Stettler, R., Moores, S.L., Pidathala, C., Müller, N., Stachulski, A., Berry, N.G., Rossignol, J.F., Hemphill, A., 2005, In vitro efficacies of nitazoxanide and other thiazolides against *Neospora caninum* tachyzoites reveal antiparasitic activity independent of the nitro group. Antimicrob Agents Chemother 49, 3715-3723.
Ferre, I., Aduriz, G., Del-Pozo, I., Regidor-Cerrillo, J., Atxaerandio, R., Collantes-Fernàndez, E., Hurtado, A., Ugarte-Garagalza, C., Ortega-Mora, L.M., 2005, Detection of *Neospora caninum* in the semen and blood of naturally infected bulls. Theriogenology 63, 1504-1518.
Ferroglio, E., Guiso, P., Pasino, M., Accossato, A., Trisciuoglio, A., 2005, Antibodies to *Neospora caninum* in stray cats from north Italy. Vet Parasitol 131, 31-34.
Ferroglio, E., Wambwa, E., Castiello, M., Trisciuoglio, A., Prouteau, A., Pradere, E., Ndungu, S., De Meneghi, D., 2003, Antibodies to *Neospora caninum* in wild animals from Kenya, East Africa. Vet Parasitol 118, 43-49.

Furr, M., Kennedy, T., 2000, Cerebrospinal fluid and blood concentrations of toltrazuril 5% suspension in the horse after oral dosing. Vet Ther 1, 123-132.

Gondim, L.F., 2006, Neospora caninum in wildlife. Trends Parasitol 22, 247-252.

Gondim, L.F., Gao, L., McAllister, M.M., 2002, Improved production of Neospora caninum oocysts, cyclical oral transmission between dogs and cattle, and in vitro isolation from oocysts. J Parasitol 88, 1159-1163.

Gondim, L.F., McAllister, M.M., Anderson-Sprecher, R.C., Björkman, C., Lock, T.F., Firkins, L.D., Gao, L., Fischer, W.R., 2004, Transplacental transmission and abortion in cows administered Neospora caninum oocysts. J Parasitol 90, 1394-1400.

Gondim, L.F., McAllister, M.M., Pitt, W.C., Zemlicka, D.E., 2004, Coyotes (Canis latrans) are definitive hosts of Neospora caninum. Int J Parasitol 34, 159-161.

Gottstein, B., Eperon, S., Dai, W.J., Cannas, A., Hemphill, A., Greif, G., 2001, Efficacy of toltrazuril and ponazuril against experimental Neospora caninum infection in mice. Parasitol Res 87, 43-48.

Gottstein, B., Razmi, G.R., Ammann, P., Sager, H., Müller, N., 2005, Toltrazuril treatment to control diaplacental Neospora caninum transmission in experimentally infected pregnant mice. Parasitology 130, 41-48.

Greif, G., 2000, Immunity to coccidiosis after treatment with toltrazuril. Parasitol Res 86, 787-790.

Haerdi, C., Haessig, M., Sager, H., Greif, G., Staubli, D., Gottstein, B., 2006, Humoral immune reaction of newborn calves congenitally infected with Neospora caninum and experimentally treated with toltrazuril. Parasitol Res 99, 534-540.

Haldorson, G.J., Mathison, B.A., Wenberg, K., Conrad, P.A., Dubey, J.P., Trees, A.J., Yamane, I., Baszler, T.V., 2005, Immunization with native surface protein NcSRS2 induces a Th2 immune response and reduces congenital Neospora caninum transmission in mice. Int J Parasitol 35, 1407-1415.

Haldorson, G.J., Stanton, J.B., Mathison, B.A., Suarez, C.E., Baszler, T.V., 2006, Neospora caninum: antibodies directed against tachyzoite surface protein NcSRS2 inhibit parasite attachment and invasion of placental trophoblasts in vitro. Exp Parasitol 112, 172-178.

Harder, A., Haberkorn, A., 1989, Possible mode of action of toltrazuril: studies on two Eimeria species and mammalian and Ascaris suum enzymes. Parasitol Res 76, 8-12.

Häsler, B., Regula, G., Stark, K.D., Sager, H., Gottstein, B., Reist, M., 2006, Financial analysis of various strategies for the control of Neospora caninum in dairy cattle in Switzerland. Prev Vet Med 77, 230-253.

Hässig, M., Sager, H., Reitt, K., Ziegler, D., Strabel, D., Gottstein, B., 2003, Neospora caninum in sheep: a herd case report. Vet Parasitol 117, 213-220.

Hemphill, A., Fuchs, N., Sonda, S., Hehl, A., 1999, The antigenic composition of Neospora caninum. Int J Parasitol 29, 1175-1188.

Hemphill, A., Gottstein, B., Kaufmann, H., 1996, Adhesion and invasion of bovine endothelial cells by Neospora caninum. Parasitology 112 (Pt 2), 183-197.

Ho, M.S., Barr, B.C., Tarantal, A.F., Lai, L.T., Hendrickx, A.G., Marsh, A.E., Sverlow, K.W., Packham, A.E., Conrad, P.A., 1997, Detection of Neospora from tissues of experimentally infected rhesus macaques by PCR and specific DNA probe hybridization. J Clin Microbiol 35, 1740-1745.

Hotta, C., Fujimaki, H., Yoshinari, M., Nakazawa, M., Minami, M., 2006, The delivery of an antigen from the endocytic compartment into the cytosol for cross-presentation is restricted to early immature dendritic cells. Immunology 117, 97-107.

Innes, E.A., Andrianarivo, A.G., Björkman, C., Williams, D.J., Conrad, P.A., 2002, Immune responses to *Neospora caninum* and prospects for vaccination. Trends Parasitol 18, 497-504.

Innes, E.A., Wright, S., Bartley, P., Maley, S., Macaldowie, C., Esteban-Redondo, I., Buxton, D., 2005, The host-parasite relationship in bovine neosporosis. Vet Immunol Immunopathol 108, 29-36.

Innes, E.A., Wright, S.E., Maley, S., Rae, A., Schock, A., Kirvar, E., Bartley, P., Hamilton, C., Carey, I.M., Buxton, D., 2001, Protection against vertical transmission in bovine neosporosis. Int J Parasitol 31, 1523-1534.

Iwasaki, A., Medzhitov, R., 2004, Toll-like receptor control of the adaptive immune responses. Nat Immunol 5, 987-995.

Kang, S.W., Kweon, C.H., Lee, E.H., Choe, S.E., Jung, S.C., Quyen, D.V., 2008, The differentiation of transcription between tachyzoites and bradyzoites of *in vitro* cultured *Neospora caninum*. Parasitol Res 103, 1011-1018.

Kano, R., Masukata, Y., Omata, Y., Kobayashi, Y., Maeda, R., Saito, A., 2005, Relationship between type 1/type 2 immune responses and occurrence of vertical transmission in BALB/c mice infected with *Neospora caninum*. Vet Parasitol 129, 159-164.

Kaufmann, H., Yamage, M., Roditi, I., Dobbelaere, D., Dubey, J.P., Holmdahl, O.J., Trees, A., Gottstein, B., 1996, Discrimination of *Neospora caninum* from *Toxoplasma gondii* and other apicomplexan parasites by hybridization and PCR. Mol Cell Probes 10, 289-297.

Kim, J.T., Park, J.Y., Seo, H.S., Oh, H.G., Noh, J.W., Kim, J.H., Kim, D.Y., Youn, H.J., 2002, In vitro antiprotozoal effects of artemisinin on *Neospora caninum*. Vet Parasitol 103, 53-63.

Koiwai, M., Hamaoka, T., Haritani, M., Shimizu, S., Tsutsui, T., Eto, M., Yamane, I., 2005, Seroprevalence of *Neospora caninum* in dairy and beef cattle with reproductive disorders in Japan. Vet Parasitol 130, 15-18.

Kritzner, S., Sager, H., Blum, J., Krebber, R., Greif, G., Gottstein, B., 2002, An explorative study to assess the efficacy of toltrazuril-sulfone (ponazuril) in calves experimentally infected with *Neospora caninum*. Ann Clin Microbiol Antimicrob 1, 4.

Kwon, H.J., Kim, J.H., Kim, M., Lee, J.K., Hwang, W.S., Kim, D.Y., 2003, Antiparasitic activity of depudecin on *Neospora caninum* via the inhibition of histone deacetylase. Vet Parasitol 112, 269-276.

Lambert, H., Hitziger, N., Dellacasa, I., Svensson, M., Barragan, A., 2006, Induction of dendritic cell migration upon *Toxoplasma gondii* infection potentiates parasite dissemination. Cell Microbiol 8, 1611-1623.

Leepin, A., Studli, A., Brun, R., Stephens, C.E., Boykin, D.W., Hemphill, A., 2008, Host cells participate in the *in vitro* effects of novel diamidine analogues against tachyzoites of the intracellular apicomplexan parasites *Neospora caninum* and *Toxoplasma gondii*. Antimicrob Agents Chemother 52, 1999-2008.

Liddell, S., Jenkins, M.C., Collica, C.M., Dubey, J.P., 1999, Prevention of vertical transfer of *Neospora caninum* in BALB/c mice by vaccination. J Parasitol 85, 1072-1075.

Liddell, S., Jenkins, M.C., Dubey, J.P., 1999, Vertical transmission of *Neospora caninum* in BALB/c mice determined by polymerase chain reaction detection. J Parasitol 85, 550-555.

Lindsay, D.S., Dubey, J.P., 1989, Evaluation of anti-coccidial drugs' inhibition of *Neospora caninum* development in cell cultures. J Parasitol 75, 990-992.

Lindsay, D.S., Dubey, J.P., 1989, *Neospora caninum* (Protozoa: apicomplexa) infections in mice. J Parasitol 75, 772-779.

Lindsay, D.S., Dubey, J.P., 1990, Effects of sulfadiazine and amprolium on *Neospora caninum* (Protozoa: Apicomplexa) infection in mice. J Parasitol 76, 177-179.

Lindsay, D.S., Dubey, J.P., Duncan, R.B., 1999, Confirmation that the dog is a definitive host for *Neospora caninum*. Vet Parasitol 82, 327-333.

Lindsay, D.S., Lenz, S.D., Cole, R.A., Dubey, J.P., Blagburn, B.L., 1995, Mouse model for central nervous system *Neospora caninum* infections. J Parasitol 81, 313-315.

Lindsay, D.S., Rippey, N.S., Cole, R.A., Parsons, L.C., Dubey, J.P., Tidwell, R.R., Blagburn, B.L., 1994, Examination of the activities of 43 chemotherapeutic agents against *Neospora caninum* tachyzoites in cultured cells. Am J Vet Res 55, 976-981.

Lindsay, D.S., Upton, S.J., Dubey, J.P., 1999, A structural study of the *Neospora caninum* oocyst. Int J Parasitol 29, 1521-1523.

Lobato, J., Silva, D.A., Mineo, T.W., Amaral, J.D., Segundo, G.R., Costa-Cruz, J.M., Ferreira, M.S., Borges, A.S., Mineo, J.R., 2006, Detection of immunoglobulin G antibodies to *Neospora caninum* in humans: high seropositivity rates in patients who are infected by human immunodeficiency virus or have neurological disorders. Clin Vaccine Immunol 13, 84-89.

Long, M.T., Baszler, T.V., 1996, Fetal loss in BALB/C mice infected with *Neospora caninum*. J Parasitol 82, 608-611.

Long, M.T., Baszler, T.V., 2000, Neutralization of maternal IL-4 modulates congenital protozoal transmission: comparison of innate versus acquired immune responses. J Immunol 164, 4768-4774.

Lopez-Gatius, F., Pabon, M., Almeria, S., 2004, *Neospora caninum* infection does not affect early pregnancy in dairy cattle. Theriogenology 62, 606-613.

Macaldowie, C., Maley, S.W., Wright, S., Bartley, P., Esteban-Redondo, I., Buxton, D., Innes, E.A., 2004, Placental pathology associated with fetal death in cattle inoculated with *Neospora caninum* by two different routes in early pregnancy. J Comp Pathol 131, 142-156.

Maley, S.W., Buxton, D., Rae, A.G., Wright, S.E., Schock, A., Bartley, P.M., Esteban-Redondo, I., Swales, C., Hamilton, C.M., Sales, J., Innes, E.A., 2003, The pathogenesis of neosporosis in pregnant cattle: inoculation at mid-gestation. J Comp Pathol 129, 186-195.

Manger, I.D., Hehl, A., Parmley, S., Sibley, L.D., Marra, M., Hillier, L., Waterston, R., Boothroyd, J., C, 1998, Expressed sequence tag analysis of the bradyzoite stage of *Toxoplasma gondii*: Identification of developmentally regulated genes. Infect Immun 66, 1623-1637.

McAllister, M.M., Björkman, C., Anderson-Sprecher, R., Rogers, D.G., 2000, Evidence of point-source exposure to *Neospora caninum* and protective immunity in a herd of beef cows. J Am Vet Med Assoc 217, 881-887.

McAllister, M.M., Dubey, J.P., Lindsay, D.S., Jolley, W.R., Wills, R.A., McGuire, A.M., 1998, Dogs are definitive hosts of *Neospora caninum*. Int J Parasitol 28, 1473-1478.

McCann, C.M., McAllister, M.M., Gondim, L.F., Smith, R.F., Cripps, P.J., Kipar, A., Williams, D.J., Trees, A.J., 2007, *Neospora caninum* in cattle: experimental infection with oocysts can result in exogenous transplacental infection, but not endogenous transplacental infection in the subsequent pregnancy. Int J Parasitol 37, 1631-1639.

McCann, C.M., Vyse, A.J., Salmon, R.L., Thomas, D., Williams, D.J., McGarry, J.W., Pebody, R., Trees, A.J., 2008, Lack of Serologic Evidence of *Neospora caninum* in Humans, England. Emerg Infect Dis 14, 978-980.

McKee, A.S., Dzierszinski, F., Boes, M., Roos, D.S., Pearce, E.J., 2004, Functional inactivation of immature dendritic cells by the intracellular parasite *Toxoplasma gondii*. J Immunol 173, 2632-2640.

Mercier, C., Lecordier, L., Darcy, F., Deslee, D., Murray, A., Tourvieille, B., Maes, P., Capron, A., Cesbron-Delauw, M.F., 1993, Molecular characterization of a dense granule antigen (Gra 2) associated with the network of the parasitophorous vacuole in *Toxoplasma gondii*. Mol Biochem Parasitol 58, 71-82.

Miller, C., Quinn, H., Ryce, C., Reichel, M.P., Ellis, J.T., 2005, Reduction in transplacental transmission of *Neospora caninum* in outbred mice by vaccination. Int J Parasitol 35, 821-828.

Morein, B., Abusugra, I., Blomqvist, G., 2002, Immunity in neonates. Vet Immunol Immunopathol 87, 207-213.

Müller, N., Sager, H., Hemphill, A., Mehlhorn, H., Heydorn, A.O., Gottstein, B., 2001, Comparative molecular investigation of Nc5-PCR amplicons from *Neospora caninum* NC-1 and *Hammondia heydorni*-Berlin-1996. Parasitol Res 87, 883-885.

Müller, N., Zimmermann, V., Hentrich, B., Gottstein, B., 1996, Diagnosis of *Neospora caninum* and *Toxoplasma gondii* infection by PCR and DNA hybridization immunoassay. J Clin Microbiol 34, 2850-2852.

Münz, C., Steinman, R.M., Fujii, S., 2005, Dendritic cell maturation by innate lymphocytes: coordinated stimulation of innate and adaptive immunity. J Exp Med 202, 203-207.

Naguleswaran, A., Müller, N., Hemphill, A., 2003, *Neospora caninum* and *Toxoplasma gondii*: a novel adhesion/invasion assay reveals distinct differences in tachyzoite-host cell interactions. Exp Parasitol 104, 149-158.

Nam, H.W., Kang, S.W., Choi, W.Y., 1998, Antibody reaction of human anti-*Toxoplasma gondii* positive and negative sera with *Neospora caninum* antigens. Korean J Parasitol 36, 269-275.

Nishikawa, Y., Inoue, N., Makala, L., Nagasawa, H., 2003, A role for balance of interferon-gamma and interleukin-4 production in protective immunity against *Neospora caninum* infection. Vet Parasitol 116, 175-184.

Nishikawa, Y., Tragoolpua, K., Inoue, N., Makala, L., Nagasawa, H., Otsuka, H., Mikami, T., 2001, In the absence of endogenous gamma interferon, mice acutely infected with *Neospora caninum* succumb to a lethal immune response characterized by inactivation of peritoneal macrophages. Clin Diagn Lab Immunol 8, 811-816.

Omata, Y., Nidaira, M., Kano, R., Kobayashi, Y., Koyama, T., Furuoka, H., Maeda, R., Matsui, T., Saito, A., 2004, Vertical transmission of *Neospora caninum* in BALB/c mice in both acute and chronic infection. Vet Parasitol 121, 323-328.

Patitucci, A.N., Alley, M.R., Jones, B.R., Charleston, W.A., 1997, Protozoal encephalomyelitis of dogs involving *Neospora caninum* and *Toxoplasma gondii* in New Zealand. N Z Vet J 45, 231-235.

Payne, S., Ellis, J., 1996, Detection of *Neospora caninum* DNA by the polymerase chain reaction. Int J Parasitol 26, 347-351.

Perl, S., Harrus, S., Satuchne, C., Yakobson, B., Haines, D., 1998, Cutaneous neosporosis in a dog in Israel. Vet Parasitol 79, 257-261.

Peters, M., Lutkefels, E., Heckeroth, A.R., Schares, G., 2001, Immunohistochemical and ultrastructural evidence for *Neospora caninum* tissue cysts in skeletal muscles of naturally infected dogs and cattle. Int J Parasitol 31, 1144-1148.

Piergili Fioretti, D., Pasquali, P., Diaferia, M., Mangili, V., Rosignoli, L., 2003, *Neospora caninum* infection and congenital transmission: serological and parasitological study of cows up to the fourth gestation. J Vet Med B Infect Dis Vet Public Health 50, 399-404.

Piergili Fioretti, D., Rosignoli, L., Ricci, G., Moretti, A., Pasquali, P., Polidori, G.A., 2000, *Neospora caninum* infection in a clinically healthy calf: parasitological study and serological follow-up. J Vet Med B Infect Dis Vet Public Health 47, 47-53.

Pinheiro, A.M., Costa, S.L., Freire, S.M., Almeida, M.A., Tardy, M., El Bacha, R., Costa, M.F., 2006, Astroglial cells in primary culture: a valid model to study *Neospora caninum* infection in the CNS. Vet Immunol Immunopathol 113, 243-247.

Quinn, H.E., Ellis, J.T., Smith, N.C., 2002, *Neospora caninum*: a cause of immune-mediated failure of pregnancy? Trends Parasitol 18, 391-394.

Quinn, H.E., Miller, C.M., Ellis, J.T., 2004, The cell-mediated immune response to *Neospora caninum* during pregnancy in the mouse is associated with a bias towards production of interleukin-4. Int J Parasitol 34, 723-732.

Quinn, H.E., Miller, C.M., Ryce, C., Windsor, P.A., Ellis, J.T., 2002, Characterization of an outbred pregnant mouse model of Neospora caninum infection. J Parasitol 88, 691-696.

Ramamoorthy, S., Duncan, R., Lindsay, D.S., Sriranganathan, N., 2007, Optimization of the use of C57BL/6 mice as a laboratory animal model for Neospora caninum vaccine studies. Vet Parasitol 145, 253-259.

Ramamoorthy, S., Lindsay, D.S., Schurig, G.G., Boyle, S.M., Duncan, R.B., Vemulapalli, R., Sriranganathan, N., 2006, Vaccination with gamma-irradiated Neospora caninum tachyzoites protects mice against acute challenge with N. caninum. J Eukaryot Microbiol 53, 151-156.

Ramamoorthy, S., Sriranganathan, N., Lindsay, D.S., 2005, Gerbil model of acute neosporosis. Vet Parasitol 127, 111-114.

Reis e Sousa, C., Hieny, S., Scharton-Kersten, T., Jankovic, D., Charest, H., Germain, R.N., Sher, A., 1997, In vivo microbial stimulation induces rapid CD40 ligand-independent production of interleukin 12 by dendritic cells and their redistribution to T cell areas. J Exp Med 186, 1819-1829.

Rettigner, C., De Meerschman, F., Focant, C., Vanderplasschen, A., Losson, B., 2004, The vertical transmission following the reactivation of a Neospora caninum chronic infection does not seem to be due to an alteration of the systemic immune response in pregnant CBA/Ca mice. Parasitology 128, 149-160.

Rettigner, C., Leclipleux, T., Do Meerschman, F., Focant, C., Losson, B., 2004, Survival, immune responses and tissue cyst production in outbred (Swiss white) and inbred (CBA/Ca) strains of mice experimentally infected with Neospora caninum tachyzoites. Vet Res 35, 225-232.

Ritter, D.M., Kerlin, R., Sibert, G., Brake, D., 2002, Immune factors influencing the course of infection with Neospora caninum in the murine host. J Parasitol 88, 271-280.

Rizzi, M., Gerloni, M., Srivastava, A.S., Wheeler, M.C., Schuler, K., Carrier, E., Zanetti, M., 2005, In utero DNA immunisation. Immunity over tolerance in fetal life. Vaccine 23, 4273-4282.

Romero, J.J., Perez, E., Frankena, K., 2004, Effect of a killed whole Neospora caninum tachyzoite vaccine on the crude abortion rate of Costa Rican dairy cows under field conditions. Vet Parasitol 123, 149-159.

Sager, H., Fischer, I., Furrer, K., Strasser, M., Waldvogel, A., Boerlin, P., Audige, L., Gottstein, B., 2001, A Swiss case-control study to assess Neospora caninum-associated bovine abortions by PCR, histopathology and serology. Vet Parasitol 102, 1-15.

Sager, H., Moret, C.S., Müller, N., Staubli, D., Esposito, M., Schares, G., Hässig, M., Stark, K., Gottstein, B., 2006, Incidence of Neospora caninum and other intestinal protozoan parasites in populations of Swiss dogs. Vet Parasitol 139, 84-92.

Scanga, C.A., Aliberti, J., Jankovic, D., Tilloy, F., Bennouna, S., Denkers, E.Y., Medzhitov, R., Sher, A., 2002, Cutting edge: MyD88 is required for resistance to *Toxoplasma gondii* infection and regulates parasite-induced IL-12 production by dendritic cells. J Immunol 168, 5997-6001.

Sojka, D.K., Huang, Y.H., Fowell, D.J., 2008, Mechanisms of regulatory T-cell suppression - a diverse arsenal for a moving target. Immunology 124, 13-22.

Speer, C.A., Dubey, J.P., McAllister, M.M., Blixt, J.A., 1999, Comparative ultrastructure of tachyzoites, bradyzoites, and tissue cysts of *Neospora caninum* and *Toxoplasma gondii*. Int J Parasitol 29, 1509-1519.

Spencer, J.A., Higginbotham, M.J., Young-White, R.R., Guarino, A.J., Blagburn, B.L., 2005, *Neospora caninum*: adoptive transfer of immune lymphocytes precipitates disease in BALB/c mice. Vet Immunol Immunopathol 106, 329-333.

Steinfelder, S., Lucius, R., Greif, G., Pogonka, T., 2005, Treatment of mice with the anticoccidial drug Toltrazuril does not interfere with the development of a specific cellular intestinal immune response to *Eimeria falciformis*. Parasitol Res 97, 458-465.

Sun, C.M., Fiette, L., Tanguy, M., Leclerc, C., Lo-Man, R., 2003, Ontogeny and innate properties of neonatal dendritic cells. Blood 102, 585-591.

Tanaka, T., Nagasawa, H., Fujisaki, K., Suzuki, N., Mikami, T., 2000, Growth-inhibitory effects of interferon-gamma on *Neospora caninum* in murine macrophages by a nitric oxide mechanism. Parasitol Res 86, 768-771.

Teixeira, L., Marques, A., Meireles, C.S., Seabra, A.R., Rodrigues, D., Madureira, P., Faustino, A.M., Silva, C., Ribeiro, A., Ferreira, P., Correia da Costa, J.M., Canada, N., Vilanova, M., 2005, Characterization of the B-cell immune response elicited in BALB/c mice challenged with *Neospora caninum* tachyzoites. Immunology 116, 38-52.

Thompson, C.B., 1995, Distinct roles for the costimulatory ligands B7-1 and B7-2 in T helper cell differentiation? Cell 81, 979-982.

Thurmond, M.C., Hietala, S.K., 1996, Culling associated with *Neospora caninum* infection in dairy cows. Am J Vet Res 57, 1559-1562.

Thurmond, M.C., Hietala, S.K., 1997, Effect of *Neospora caninum* infection on milk production in first-lactation dairy cows. J Am Vet Med Assoc 210, 672-674.

Tranas, J., Heinzen, R.A., Weiss, L.M., McAllister, M.M., 1999, Serological evidence of human infection with the protozoan *Neospora caninum*. Clin Diagn Lab Immunol 6, 765-767.

Trees, A.J., Williams, D.J., 2005, Endogenous and exogenous transplacental infection in *Neospora caninum* and *Toxoplasma gondii*. Trends Parasitol 21, 558-561.

Veeraseatakul, P., Chutipongvivate, S., 2005, Major histocompatibility complex class II and co-stimulatory molecule CD80 expression in splenic dendritic cells from BALB/c mice infected with *Neospora caninum*. J Trop Med Parasitol 28, 31-38.

Venturini, M.C., Venturini, L., Bacigalupe, D., Machuca, M., Echaide, I., Basso, W., Unzaga, J.M., Di Lorenzo, C., Guglielmone, A., Jenkins, M.C., Dubey, J.P., 1999, *Neospora caninum* infections in bovine foetuses and dairy cows with abortions in Argentina. Int J Parasitol 29, 1705-1708.

Vonlaufen, N., Gianinazzi, C., Müller, N., Simon, F., Björkman, C., Jungi, T.W., Leib, S.L., Hemphill, A., 2002, Infection of organotypic slice cultures from rat central nervous tissue with Neospora caninum: an alternative approach to study host-parasite interactions. Int J Parasitol 32, 533-542.

Vonlaufen, N., Guetg, N., Naguleswaran, A., Müller, N., Björkman, C., Schares, G., von Blumroeder, D., Ellis, J., Hemphill, A., 2004, In vitro induction of Neospora caninum bradyzoites in vero cells reveals differential antigen expression, localization, and host-cell recognition of tachyzoites and bradyzoites. Infect Immun 72, 576-583.

Vonlaufen, N., Müller, N., Keller, N., Naguleswaran, A., Bohne, W., McAllister, M.M., Björkman, C., Müller, E., Caldelari, R., Hemphill, A., 2002, Exogenous nitric oxide triggers Neospora caninum tachyzoite-to-bradyzoite stage conversion in murine epidermal keratinocyte cell cultures. Int J Parasitol 32, 1253-1265.

Williams, D.J., Guy, C.S., McGarry, J.W., Guy, F., Tasker, L., Smith, R.F., MacEachern, K., Cripps, P.J., Kelly, D.F., Trees, A.J., 2000, Neospora caninum-associated abortion in cattle: the time of experimentally-induced parasitaemia during gestation determines foetal survival. Parasitology 121 (Pt 4), 347-358.

Williams, D.J., Guy, C.S., Smith, R.F., Ellis, J., Björkman, C., Reichel, M.P., Trees, A.J., 2007, Immunization of Cattle with Live Tachyzoites of Neospora caninum Confers Protection against Fetal Death. Infect Immun 75, 1343-1348.

Williams, D.J., Trooe, A.J., 2006, Protecting babies: vaccine strategies to prevent foetopathy in Neospora caninum-infected cattle. Parasite Immunol 28, 61-07.

Wouda, W., Moen, A.R., Schukken, Y.H., 1998, Abortion risk in progeny of cows after a Neospora caninum epidemic. Theriogenology 49, 1311-1316.

Yarovinsky, F., Zhang, D., Andersen, J.F., Bannenberg, G.L., Serhan, C.N., Hayden, M.S., Hieny, S., Sutterwala, F.S., Flavell, R.A., Ghosh, S., Sher, A., 2005, TLR11 activation of dendritic cells by a protozoan profilin-like protein. Science 308, 1626-1629.

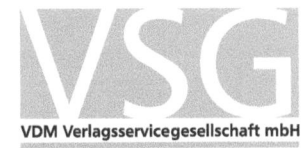

Die VDM Verlagsservicegesellschaft sucht für wissenschaftliche Verlage abgeschlossene und herausragende

## Dissertationen, Habilitationen, Diplomarbeiten, Master Theses, Magisterarbeiten usw.

für die kostenlose Publikation als Fachbuch.

Sie verfügen über eine Arbeit, die hohen inhaltlichen und formalen Ansprüchen genügt, und haben Interesse an einer honorarvergüteten Publikation?

Dann senden Sie bitte erste Informationen über sich und Ihre Arbeit per Email an *info@vdm-vsg.de*.

**Sie erhalten kurzfristig unser Feedback!**

VDM Verlagsservicegesellschaft mbH
Dudweiler Landstr. 99      Telefon  +49 681 3720 174
D - 66123 Saarbrücken      Fax      +49 681 3720 1749
**www.vdm-vsg.de**

Die VDM Verlagsservicegesellschaft mbH vertritt

 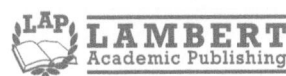 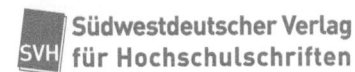

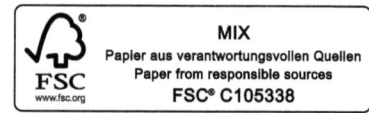

Printed by Books on Demand GmbH, Norderstedt / Germany